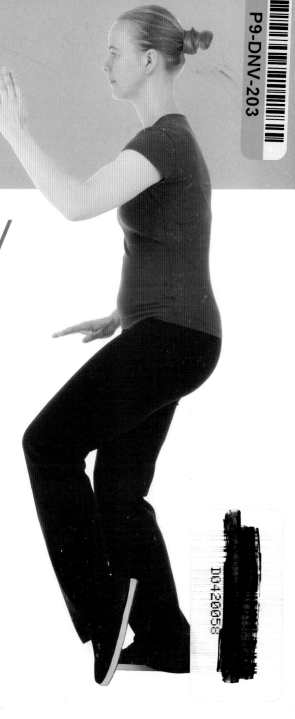

# TAI CHI
## for every body

### EASY LOW-IMPACT EXERCISES FOR EVERY AGE

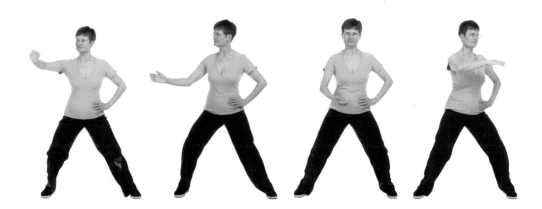

Eva **and** Karel Koskuba

**Reader's Digest**

THE READER'S DIGEST ASSOCIATION, INC.
PLEASANTVILLE, NY/MONTREAL/SYDNEY/LONDON/SINGAPORE

A READER'S DIGEST BOOK
Published by The Reader's Digest Association in arrangement with Tucker Slingsby Ltd.

Library of Congress Cataloging-in-Publication Data

Koskuba, Eva.
  Tai Chi for every body : easy low-impact exercises for every age /
    Eva and Karel Koskuba.
    p. cm.
  Includes index.
  ISBN 13: 978-0-7621-0684-4
  ISBN 10: 0-7621-0684-0
1. Tai Chi.  I. Koskuba, Karel.  II. Title.
GV504.K67 2007
613.7'148--dc22

                                                2006041761

FOR TUCKER SLINGSBY
Editorial: Sally Harding, Nicole Foster, Del Tucker
Design: Robert Mathias
Flo-mos and design production: Steve Rowling
Production: Harriet Maxwell
Photography: Andrew Sydenham
Index: Marie Lorimer

FOR READER'S DIGEST
U.S. Project Editor: Kimberly Casey
Canadian Project Editor: Pamela Johnson
Copy Editor: Barbara Booth
Associate Art Director: George McKeon
Executive Editor, Trade Publishing: Dolores York
President & Publisher, Trade Publishing: Harold Clarke

**A NOTE TO OUR READERS**
It is always advisable to check with your doctor before starting an exercise program. Consult your doctor about any symptoms that may require diagnosis or medical attention. Pregnant women are particularly advised to consult their doctor before starting Tai Chi practice. While the advice and information in this book are believed to be accurate and the exercises have been devised to avoid strain, neither the authors, the publisher, nor the copyright holder can accept any legal responsibility for any injury sustained while doing the poses and exercises in this book.

Address any comments about *Tai Chi for Every Body* to:
The Reader's Digest Association, Inc., Adult Trade Publishing, Reader's Digest Road,
Pleasantville, NY 10570-7000

For Reader's Digest products and information, visit our websites:
www.rd.com (in the United States)   www.readersdigest.ca (in Canada)
www.readersdigest.com.au (in Australia)   www.readersdigest.com.nz (in New Zealand)
www.readersdigest.co.uk (in the United Kingdom)   www.rdasia.com (in Singapore)

Manufactured in China

3  5  7  9  10  8  6  4  2

# CONTENTS

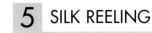
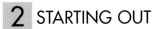
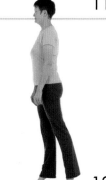
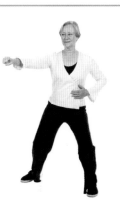

# TAI CHI IS FOR EVERYBODY

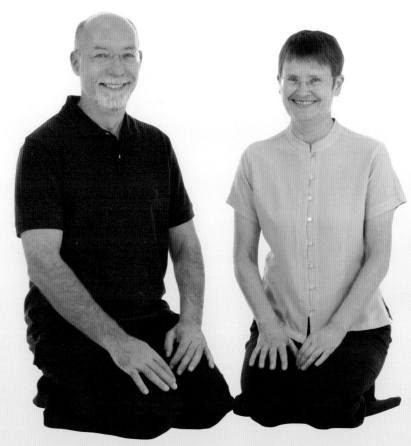

*Development in science is beyond boundary, so is practicing Tai Chi Chuan; one could never exhaust all its beauty and benefits in one's lifetime.*

—MASTER CHEN XIAOWANG,
19TH-GENERATION CHEN PATRIARCH

Throughout Chinese history there have been many holistic, therapeutic, martial, and spiritual systems. Judging by the number of people who practice it, Tai Chi is the most successful of them all. Originally a martial art accessible to only a few, it has now become a worldwide health phenomenon.

The popularity of Tai Chi is partially due to its accessibility. It doesn't require any special clothes, equipment, or place to practice. And it doesn't matter what age you are or what your fitness level is. Everybody can learn Tai Chi and reap its benefits. Tai Chi is also suitable for today's busy lifestyle. It is excellent for getting rid of stress, it is gentle on the body, yet it can be as vigorous as one wants it to be.

People take up Tai Chi for many different reasons. It can cultivate calm and tranquillity, increase strength and vitality, maintain health, or develop martial arts skills. If you wish, Tai Chi can simply be an occasional hobby or a pleasant way to unwind and relax after a busy day. Once you've started, it might, if you are so inclined, become a passionate pursuit of perfection—perfection of movement, of awareness, of being.

This book is designed to teach simple exercises to improve your health, but it can also be used to embark on a lifelong journey of self-discovery. For all of its apparent simplicity, when practiced regularly and integrated into daily life, Tai Chi has the power to enhance emotional and spiritual needs and transform lives.

Concentration is the key to discovering the secrets of Tai Chi. Are you aware of your posture as you read this? Try scanning your body for any tension. You can probably feel your body realigning and becoming more at ease. No matter how small the sensation, it is better than nothing. It's time to start practicing Tai Chi!

—Karel and Eva Koskuba

# CHAPTER 1

# About Tai Chi

In this chapter, you will discover the art of Tai Chi—where it came from, how it works, and why it is good for you. Find out how Tai Chi can fit into your everyday life, and learn the strategies to carry it out.

*Tai Chi is born out of infinity.*

—FROM THE TAI CHI *Classics*

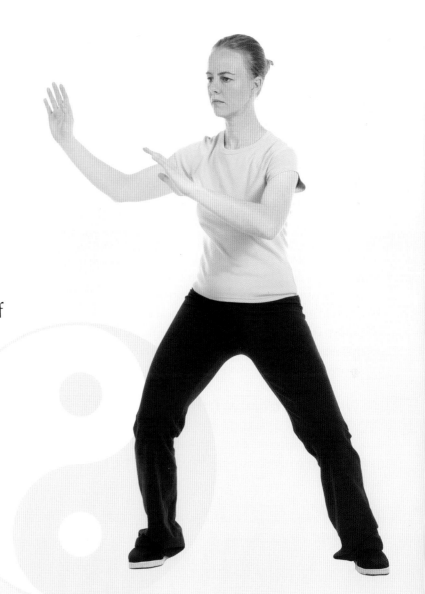

# TAI CHI FOR WELL-BEING

Tai Chi was developed in the seventeenth century in China as a martial art. Today, however, it is practiced all around the world as a simple, gentle, beneficial fitness regime.

This book covers all the exercises you need to learn to practice Tai Chi for general physical health and mental and emotional well-being. Following through, chapter by chapter, will give you a good grounding in Tai Chi. You will then be able to take this regimen to any level you wish.

If a gentle exercise routine is what you're after, then this book provides all you'll need. If you want to progress further, it also gives you tips for continual improvement of your practice. If you're looking to use Tai Chi for self-defense, then the essentials you'll learn here will prepare you well for more advanced lessons.

## How you practice Tai Chi

Tai Chi exercises consist of slow, continuous, and flowing movements. They are practiced in a calm manner and with unhurried breathing. Tai Chi trains the mind and body together. The aim is to achieve effortless power. The first step toward this is the cultivation of relaxation and a strong, steady, and rooted physical and emotional grounding. This is why Tai Chi is sometimes called "meditation in motion."

The Tai Chi beginners exercise routines contained in this book are Silk Reeling and the Tai Chi Form. The Form is a series of fluid, graceful movements, and it is the main training exercise. Silk Reeling is a number of body-twisting movements used as a preparation for practicing the Form.

All Tai Chi exercises are performed standing. Gentle, slow, soft, and contemplative, they are suitable for all fitness levels, body shapes, and age groups. They require no special clothing or equipment and can be done anywhere.

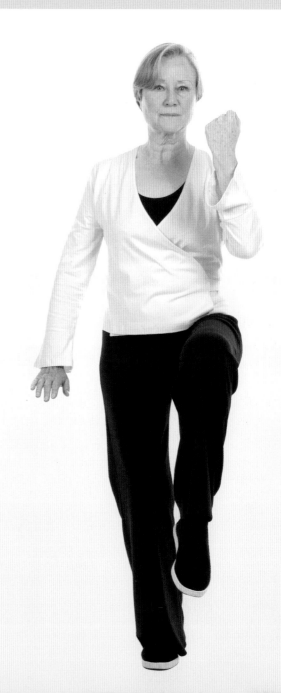

### BENEFITS OF TAI CHI

Practicing Tai Chi will improve your whole quality of life, from better health to greater physical and emotional confidence. It will increase your energy level, alertness, strength, and flexibility. Students of Tai Chi of all ages also notice greatly improved coordination and balance, which impact everyday life in many ways—from putting on socks and shoes to tackling daily chores and playing sports. (See pages 129–136 for more about Tai Chi and health.)

# How Tai Chi works

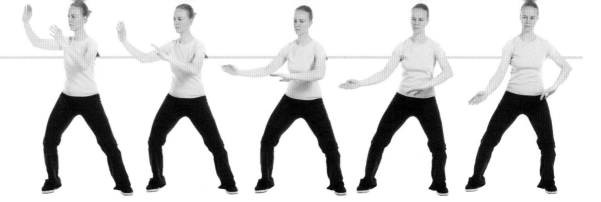

The theory behind Tai Chi is rooted in Chinese culture and based on texts called the Tai Chi *Classics* that were written by past Tai Chi masters.

The first stage in Tai Chi training is to cultivate what the Chinese call *chi*, which is most closely translated as intrinsic energy. Everyone has *chi*, but most people don't know how to use it. Through training to relax, concentrate, and use minimal physical effort, Tai Chi students learn how to "use *chi*" to gain effortless movement.

## Tonic and phasic muscles

The best way to understand how Tai Chi training works is to understand the difference between tonic and phasic muscles. You are not really aware of your tonic muscles: They balance and support your posture, stabilizing your body against the pull of gravity; they are not under your conscious control, and their use is effortless. Phasic muscles are muscles you use to move, and you have conscious control over them. You can contract and relax these muscles at will; using them requires effort. Tonic muscles are always working, whether you are moving or not.

When first practicing Tai Chi, the emphasis is on learning correct posture using only tonic muscles to support your body, even in movement. The trick is to

### THE TAI CHI ROAD MAP

- Relaxation is the prerequisite.
- Concentration/mental focus is the means.
- Posture, coordination, breathing are the steps.
- Internal power is the goal.

move slowly and fluidly from one position to the next, as if you are being pushed. To do this, you will need to consciously relax your phasic muscles. This first stage of Tai Chi is the one covered in this book and is the one that gives the most health benefits.

## Tai Chi theory and *chi*

While studying Tai Chi, you will come across constant references to being relaxed, not tensing muscles, and even not using muscles. The old Tai Chi masters were not interested in anatomical accuracy and probably knew very little about anatomy as we understand it today.

They were interested in functional explanations that students could follow in their studies. As far as they were concerned, muscle effort is a conscious activity, which is more or less the way we think about it in our everyday life, too. They were not aware of the tonic muscles that stabilize our body against gravity. In their line of thinking, our ability to stand without any obvious effort was due to *chi*, like anything else that is outside our awareness (for example, digestion, blood circulation, and so on). Thus, their advice to relax all muscles and "use your *chi*" is really advice to relax all muscles that we can consciously relax, which we now know are the phasic muscles.

### YIN AND YANG

The terms "Tai Chi" and "Tai Chi Chuan" are used interchangeably. Tai Chi means "supreme ultimate," and Chuan means "boxing" or "fist." Tai Chi is also the name of the Yin Yang diagram, which precedes the birth of Tai Chi as an exercise regime. In Chinese culture the world has traditionally been seen as the interplay of two principles—the Yin and the Yang—and Tai Chi Chuan has always been regarded as the embodiment of these two principles.

In the Tai Chi diagram the white represents Yang, which is rising, and the dark area represents Yin, which is descending. The shapes illustrate how when Yang reaches its peak, it gives rise to Yin; the Yin, in turn, when it reaches its maximum, gives rise to Yang. The two small circles represent Yin within Yang and Yang within Yin to indicate the idea that the two cannot be separated (see also page 16).

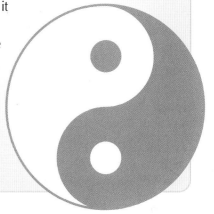

# Tai Chi in everyday life

When you start practicing Tai Chi, you will be surprised at how quickly your body awareness improves. This improvement will continue as long as you keep practicing, and eventually it will show in your physical and mental abilities. This applies to all age groups. After a period of Tai Chi training, an elderly woman who had always struggled lifting a saddle onto her horse found she could do it easily because of subtle shifts in the way she used her body.

Tai Chi students find that their increased body awareness enables them to practice anywhere without looking as if they are practicing. Everyday movement becomes Tai Chi practice. It is not something that Tai Chi students have to force themselves to do; it is something they enjoy doing.

If you watch a cat, for example, you'll notice that although it doesn't practice Tai Chi, it remains supple, agile, and strong—and it looks like it enjoys its body moving. When you practice Tai Chi, you eventually achieve a state where the movement itself becomes enjoyable and sensuous. With more practice, this sense will carry over to your normal movement in everyday life. You start moving like a cat—but hopefully not on all fours!

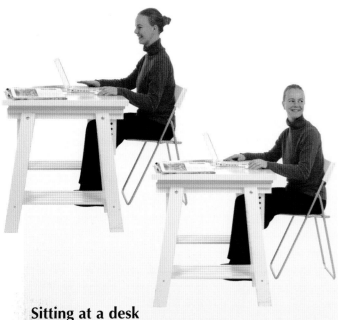

### Sitting at a desk
Your Tai Chi lessons will teach you a balanced, relaxed posture that you can apply sitting at your desk working. After you have practiced Tai Chi for a while, like this Tai Chi teacher, you will even remain balanced, supple, and straight when you turn to look over your shoulder in a sitting position.

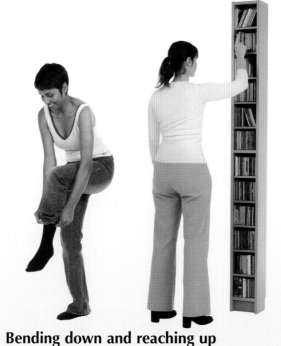

### Bending down and reaching up
These Tai Chi students use their Tai Chi practice in everyday life by keeping a strong, steady, rooted, relaxed posture at all times. When bending over, the student on the left stays firmly balanced. When reaching up for objects, the student on the right keeps her shoulders down and relaxed, legs solid, and spine straight.

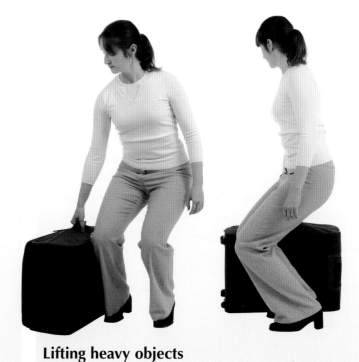

### Lifting heavy objects
We are all at risk of back injury when lifting heavy objects. A Tai Chi student finds it easy to keep a strong, straight back and uses muscles in an effortless way that protects the back from strain.

# Guidelines for practicing Tai Chi

The first thing to realize is that your main task when learning Tai Chi is to train your mind, not your body. Follow the instructions for the movements as best you can, but pay particular attention to the guidelines for relaxing and staying aware of the sensations in your body.

## How much and how often

It pays to establish a regular routine. Practicing Tai Chi a little every day is better than practicing a lot infrequently. It is also easier to carry on practicing if you have a regular routine. Try practicing only for as long as your concentration lasts. If you get bored or can't concentrate, stop for the day.

## Pain is not necessary

Pain is distracting. Remember, you are training your mind—if the pain in your legs or arms distracts you, you can't concentrate, so stop practicing or change to another posture. You should never feel pain in your joints, so if you do, stop practicing.

## Get someone to correct your postures

At the very beginning of the Tai Chi learning process, it's a good idea not to worry about whether you are positioned in precisely the way given in the instructions. First you need to relax and settle into the practice and movements. After a while you should get someone to check whether you are standing and moving in the positions pictured in the book. Having someone check you will save a lot of time, and eventually you will be able to feel for yourself whether you are assuming the correct postures or not.

## Standing practice

Standing practice, or Zhan Zhuang, is used in Tai Chi to correct posture and for relaxation. You will learn how to do this in Chapter 2 (see pages 21 and 22). You should do standing practice regularly and increase the amount of time spent on it gradually until you can do 20 minutes every day. Zhan Zhuang trains your awareness, and students who stand regularly make the best progress.

## TIPS FOR PRACTICE

Before you start on any of the Tai Chi exercises in the book, bear in mind these general points:

- The less strength you use, the better.

- There should be no strain felt anywhere in your body or mind as a result of the exercises.

- Try to keep a balanced and relaxed posture throughout. If there is a conflict between doing an exercise correctly and keeping a balanced posture, choose the balanced posture! If the posture is not balanced, chances are the exercise should be performed differently anyway—check it again.

- Pay attention to the way your body moves and the associated sensations. Only when moving with awareness can you change the ingrained patterns of movement.

- Keep your breathing even and comfortable.

### Warming up
The calf-stretching exercise on the left is one of the many simple warm-up exercises you should do before starting your Tai Chi movements (see Chapter 3 on pages 23–38).

9

# How to use this book

The Tai Chi lessons in this book should be followed in the order they are given. That means you should do the lessons in Chapter 2 before moving on to the following chapter, and so on. Pay special attention to the tip and information boxes.

## Getting into it

Chapter 2 (Starting Out) explains how your balance works and how to achieve a good standing posture. It also teaches you how to begin to relax your body with a standing practice called Zhan Zhuang. Chapter 3 gives warm-up exercises you should use every time you start practicing Tai Chi. Basic Tai Chi stances and hand positions, plus how to perform simple Tai Chi Stepping, are covered in Chapter 4.

## Learning the movements

Chapter 5 provides how-to steps for learning Silk Reeling moves, the basis of all Tai Chi movement. Learning the Form is broken down into stages—Chapter 6 teaches some of the main body positions found in the Form that you can practice as static exercises, Chapter 7 describes in detail each individual exercise of the Form, and Chapter 8 illustrates the Form as one flowing series of moves.

## Perfecting your Tai Chi

Those who want to continue to improve their performance of the Tai Chi movements learned in this book can delve into the theory of how to perfect Tai Chi movement and power in Chapter 9.

## Benefits of Tai Chi

Chapter 10 outlines in more detail all the health benefits of Tai Chi and provides two simple exercises anyone can do to improve strength and balance.

## Clothes, equipment, and location

There is no need for special clothes for Tai Chi. All you need is a comfortable outfit that does not restrict your movement and some comfortable shoes (unless you can do it barefoot). Tai Chi teachers sometimes give demonstrations wearing traditional Chinese silk suits. The hang of the silk garments gives the wearer an enhanced sense of movement and balance and highlights their gracefulness, but they are not necessary for everyday Tai Chi practice.

There is also no need for any special equipment, especially when you are starting out. You can enjoy practicing Tai Chi for decades without any equipment and still not exhaust its magic.

Advanced Tai Chi, however, is sometimes performed with traditional weapons—sword, broadsword (saber), spear, and others. The reason for choosing to learn weapon practice can be for enjoyment or as a supplemental strength training,

in which case the weapons are often very heavy.

The best place to practice Tai Chi is outdoors in nature. If you live in a city and don't have an outdoor space to practice in at home, use a suitable park. These days you often find people practicing in parks, and curious onlookers are becoming a thing of the past. If you prefer privacy, especially when you start out with your Tai Chi, it is just as easy to practice indoors.

CHAPTER

# 2 Starting Out

Movements in Tai Chi should be natural. This
sounds easy, but unfortunately, since stressful
and sedentary modern lifestyles create tension
and imbalances in the body, natural motion
doesn't come easily to most people.
In this chapter, we shall discover
what makes for natural posture and
movement.

*A journey of a thousand miles starts
with the first step.*

—FROM *Dao De Jing* BY LAO TZU

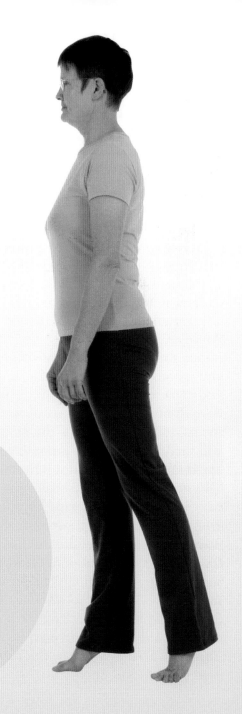

# POSTURE AND MOVEMENT

When starting out in Tai Chi, you will begin to see how the muscles that control your posture work automatically to support every movement you make—even when you think you are standing perfectly still.

*Posture is basic; movement is supported by posture at all times.*

The man pictured at right is standing in a static, well-balanced posture. The only work your muscles do when you are standing like this is to support your body against gravity. Try it and see how still you can become. Pay attention to your body as you relax in a standing position. You will notice that your muscles constantly adjust your posture to maintain balance without you consciously being involved. If you have difficulty sensing these subtle movements, stand on one leg—the movement will then become more pronounced. Even apparent stillness contains movement.

To stop these natural, small adjustments to your posture, you would have to tense your muscles. In fact, some people unknowingly store tension in their body, which, however slight, interferes with the body's natural operation. The postural muscles are designed to work against gravity, and if they are prevented from doing this, their function can become impaired. So if you release the tension, your posture will improve.

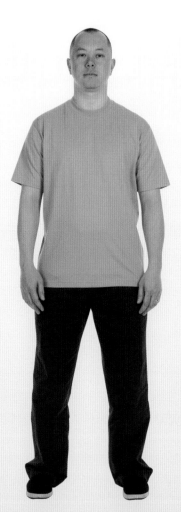

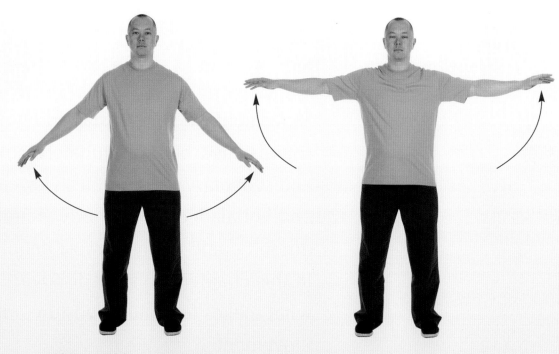

### Lifting and lowering arms

Try lifting your arms as shown above and then lowering them. Start by lifting your arms to shoulder height and holding them there for a second or two. Consciously relax your shoulders while keeping your arms at the same height. Your shoulders will probably visibly sink.

Now perform the same movement again, but this time move slowly, as if feeling your way—without stopping—through a series of static postures. Again relax your shoulders as you did before and see if there is any difference between the two actions.

Hopefully, the second time around, your arms will be more relaxed, and since you are not tense, your shoulders will not visibly sink.

# Try Stepping

To find out how posture and movement are linked, simply try Stepping forward. To see how your balance is affected as your body moves from one position to the next, first try Stepping at a normal speed and, as you move, concentrate on how your balance feels at each phase of the movement so you can recall it later.

Now try Stepping forward again, but this time move very slowly, with your feet floating slowly through space. You will probably find this more of a challenge because it puts your balance under a spotlight.

Next, when Stepping slowly, try to hold each of the eight positions for about three breaths (20 seconds). You will feel yourself gradually letting go of tension in your body. If you start to sway or wobble, hold the position for just one or two breaths and, as your balance improves, build up to a slower movement.

Once you can hold each position comfortably, move through the individual positions slowly and continuously. You should now find that you flow through the movement more smoothly, you feel relaxed, and your balance is better.

After practicing at a slow speed for a while, try Stepping at a normal speed again. Compared to your first experience, you should feel more poised and balanced, and your steps should be lighter and more agile.

> **WHY SLOW MOVEMENT IS IMPORTANT**
>
> As you hold each posture, you give your mind time to focus on improving your balance. By consciously trying to relax your muscles, you will achieve a more correct posture. Your mind will recall this muscular pattern the next time you try the movement at slow speed. Eventually you will retain improved balance and more relaxed muscles, even when moving at normal speed.

## Taking simple steps

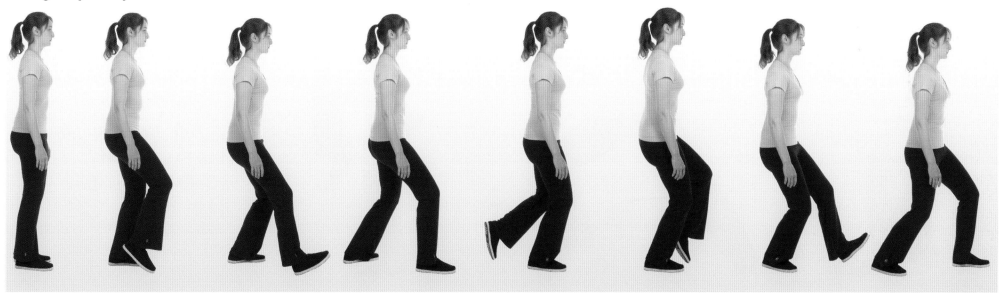

# Balance (is) everywhere

Now take a look at these Tai Chi stances. Most of us are easily aware of proper balance when we are standing upright. But when a posture is not upright, balance is more difficult to achieve.

When you bend your body away from an upright standing position, extra effort is needed to hold the posture. If this effort is felt as tension, it will interfere with effortless movement.

With practice, it is possible to find balance in most postures. To do this, try to relax into the posture and experiment with slight movements of your muscles as they guide your body into a more comfortable position. By relaxing, you are letting your body's natural reactions take over to find its own correct balance.

The more you practice being balanced, the easier it becomes and the better for your everyday life.

### White Crane Spreads Its Wings

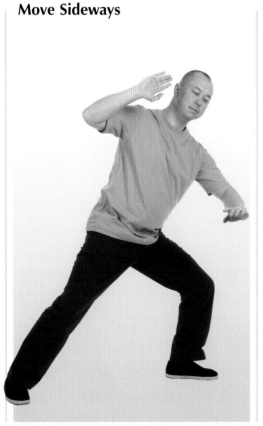

### Move Sideways

### Jin Gang Pounds Mortar

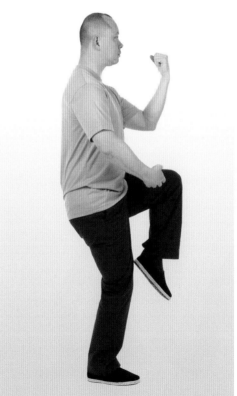

*Postural muscles support your body against the force of gravity. Sensors in your muscles, tendons, and joints send signals to your brain that help your body maintain a natural balanced posture.*

# Balance and posture

As a species, humans have not adapted perfectly to our upright posture. As a result, the postural muscles that work to balance our bodies are often not used properly. When this happens, the muscles either stop working efficiently or may even stop working altogether. This allows other muscles, less suited to the task, to take over.

One example of this is demonstrated by the seated positions below. In the one on the left, the postural muscles correctly support the torso and head; in the picture on the right, postural muscles support only the head. Over time, this incorrect posture will cause the muscles that should be supporting the torso to weaken, and when an upright posture is attempted, the muscles will ache—probably resulting in a slumped sitting posture.

Maintaining good postural balance will result in free, effortless movement. Poor use of postural muscles, which is most often the norm, results in stiffness and a sense of effort on movement. When some of the postural muscles stop participating in maintaining an upright posture, one of the important goals of Tai Chi—achieving whole-body power—becomes virtually impossible.

**Correct use of postural muscles**

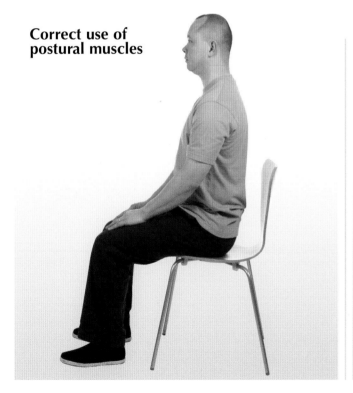

**Incorrect use of postural muscles**

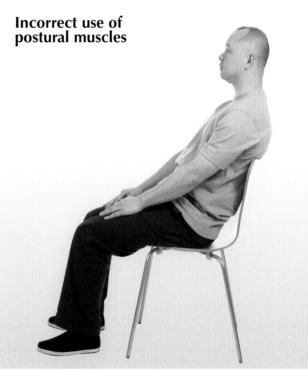

## ELIMINATING THE SENSE OF EFFORT

The first task of Tai Chi is to learn to use your postural muscles correctly, thus eliminating all sense of muscular effort. To show you how this can be achieved, try to balance a stick on the palm of your hand as shown in the picture below.

You will notice that you need to give your arm freedom to move in response to changes of the stick's position—which is impossible if you keep your arm tense. Note also how you control the outcome—keeping the stick upright—but not the individual moves. It is as if your arm has a will of its own.

This is how your postural muscles keep you upright. They act without your conscious involvement, but unlike a stick, your body contains sensors linked to the postural system that make the corrections far more immediate and precise.

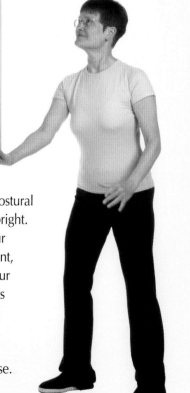

# Learning more about balance

Let's try another experiment to illustrate how your postural muscles should be working. First, hold a stick close to its base as shown below left. Keep the stick vertical and don't allow it to move—this action is "holding." Next, relax the hand and arm and balance the stick as shown below right—this action is "balancing." Try switching between these two actions a few times, and note what happens in your arm and hand as you switch.

Now see how this experiment correlates with the action of your body. First, just stand still and be aware of whether you are "holding" your body upright or whether you are "balancing" it. Then try the same as you walk.

Most of the time we "hold" our body. To "balance" the body takes concentration, which we fear will interfere with our normal activities. However, "balancing" is a very efficient way of getting in touch with the body's postural system—whether we are standing still or moving. In fact, it is only through "balancing" that we are aware of postural muscles during movement.

*Body balance is the key to the correct use of postural muscles.*

### YIN AND YANG

You can now start to understand how the two principles Yin and Yang come into Tai Chi. Any action that results from the postural muscles (not actively directed by us) is seen as Yin, and any action that results from the phasic muscles (the muscles for movement that are under our conscious control) is seen as Yang.

The first stage of training is very much Yin; this stage is characterized by slow and relaxed movement, and because the postural muscles are not under our conscious control, internal sensations known as *chi* are used to guide our practice.

The second stage is Yang and is characterized by fast movement and explosive strength. Without a clear understanding of the first stage, the second stage is difficult. That is why most of the Tai Chi you see is of the slow, relaxed variety only.

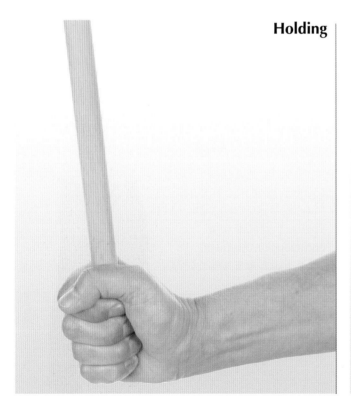

**Holding**

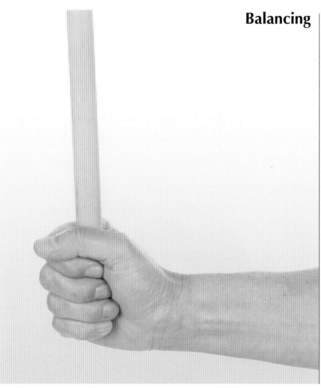

**Balancing**

# Basic Posture in focus

Basic Posture is used at the beginning of most Tai Chi exercises. It may look easy, but at first you will need a fair amount of concentration to achieve it.

To stand in Basic Posture, place your feet shoulder-width apart and parallel. The ball of the foot should feel as if it is being pulled upward and toward the heel, maintaining the foot's natural arch. Feel your toes pressing lightly into the ground. Distribute your weight evenly between the left and right foot and just in front of each heel.

Keep your knees slightly flexed and pointing in the same direction as the toes. Imagine there is a balloon between your knees and they are exerting barely perceptible pressure on it to keep it from falling.

Your pelvis should be horizontal and your weight evenly distributed across the hips. To achieve the correct vertical posture, feel the "sitting bones" sink down (releasing any tension in the lower back) and the tips of the hip bones in front floating upward.

Imagine that your rib cage is a bell hanging from your neck so that the lower front ribs sink down and the lower back ribs slide back. Feel as if your diaphragm is horizontal.

The front of the shoulders should be open and wide and the back wide. Keep the shoulder blades flat, with a feeling that the lower tips are being pulled toward the center of the lower back. There should be a feeling of space in your armpits.

The top of the head should be horizontal, the floor of the mouth relaxed, and the eyes looking forward. Feel as if your head is floating upward. Keep your spine vertical between the sinking pelvis and floating head. Feel it lengthening and relaxing.

## FOLLOW THESE GUIDELINES

Stay soft and relaxed. Sense the body's balance and relax muscles not involved in the balancing action. Feel your weight like a liquid flowing down through your legs into the ground. When trying to adjust your posture, focus on the sensations and on an image of the body area rather than its actual position. Remember, you are trying to work with postural muscles that are not under your conscious control. Use images, follow body sensations, and be patient—your posture will improve slowly over time.

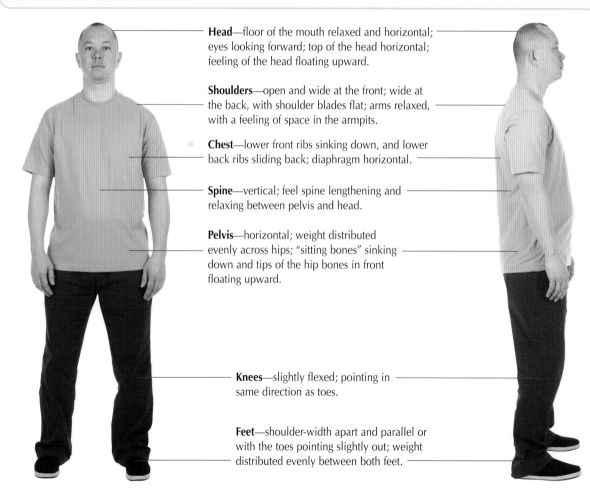

**Head**—floor of the mouth relaxed and horizontal; eyes looking forward; top of the head horizontal; feeling of the head floating upward.

**Shoulders**—open and wide at the front; wide at the back, with shoulder blades flat; arms relaxed, with a feeling of space in the armpits.

**Chest**—lower front ribs sinking down, and lower back ribs sliding back; diaphragm horizontal.

**Spine**—vertical; feel spine lengthening and relaxing between pelvis and head.

**Pelvis**—horizontal; weight distributed evenly across hips; "sitting bones" sinking down and tips of the hip bones in front floating upward.

**Knees**—slightly flexed; pointing in same direction as toes.

**Feet**—shoulder-width apart and parallel or with the toes pointing slightly out; weight distributed evenly between both feet.

# Tips to correct your posture

You need to develop an awareness of your body in space so that you can rely on this to sense whether your posture is correct or not. As you practice the postures and movements, your body awareness will improve. But to get you started, here are some tips:

At first, your sense of place and position will not be reliable, so check your posture in a mirror. If you can see a pattern with horizontal and vertical lines behind you, that is even better (a mirror facing tiles in the bathroom works well). Use these to check your body alignment such as shoulder line, body line, and head position.

When you feel your body is in the correct position (or at least an improved one), try to feel this posture without looking in the mirror. Do this for parts of the body that you can see easily. For example, after aligning your feet, try to feel their position without looking at them. Next time, try to position them using the feeling and check visually afterward.

Gradually your body awareness will improve.

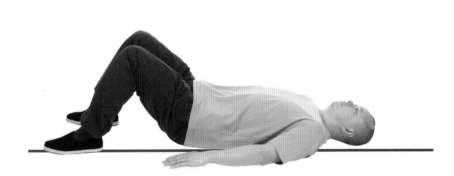

## Exercises to correct posture

If you find it difficult to sense if your posture is correct, if the tension in your back persists, or if you have an arched lower back (see right), try these two exercises.

First, lie down on the floor with your knees bent. Feel your spine relaxing into the floor. Let the lower back and the lower chest relax. After a few days of this practice (5–10 minutes at a time), add

a second exercise. Stand against a wall and pretend that you are still lying down—with the wall behind replacing the floor beneath you. Keep relaxing the spine into the "floor." After a few more days stand just next to the wall and occasionally sway back to touch the wall to feel your alignment.

Come back to these exercises later if you feel the need.

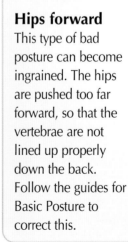

## COMMON POSTURAL PROBLEMS

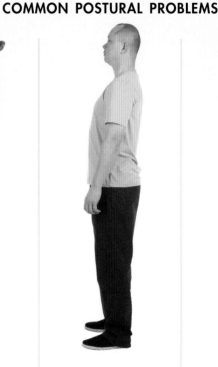

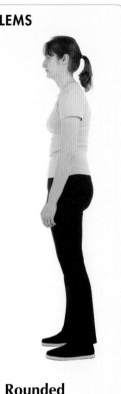

### Hips forward
This type of bad posture can become ingrained. The hips are pushed too far forward, so that the vertebrae are not lined up properly down the back. Follow the guides for Basic Posture to correct this.

### Thrust-out chest
This may result from an arched lower back. To correct, imagine a weight hanging from the back of your pelvis and a lifting at the front. Feel the skin on the back of your legs sink down and the skin on the front of your legs slide up.

### Rounded shoulders
This is a common problem. To rectify it, make sure your shoulders are wide open with your shoulder blades flat (see page 20). With practice, good posture will become automatic.

# Well-positioned feet and ankles

If you have flat feet, or a tendency toward it, you should take extra care to make sure that the arches of your feet are working properly. You can check this out by looking at the position of your ankles. To do this, stand with one foot in front of the other. Rotate the front knee from side to side and observe the position of your lower leg and ankle. When rotating inward, you may see the ankle "collapse" and see it being raised when rotating outward. Find a position where the ankle feels strong and solid and the front of the lower leg (the shinbone) points to the center of the foot. Put your weight on the foot and relax the ankle. If it collapses and moves inward, you probably need to strengthen the arch.

To strengthen your arches, use these exercises. Also, when standing in the Tai Chi Basic Posture, create a feeling in the foot as if the ball of the foot is being pulled toward the heel and the foot arch is raised.

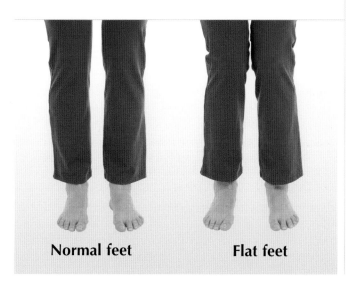

**Normal feet**          **Flat feet**

## Exercises to strengthen arches

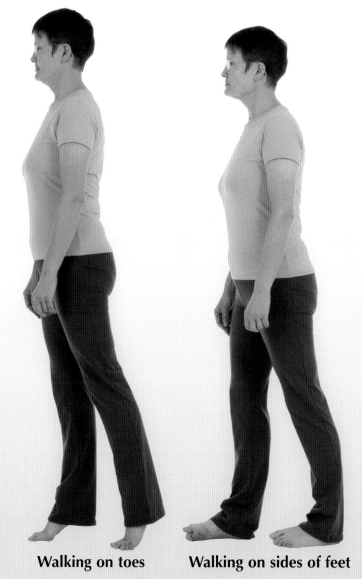

**Walking on toes**          **Walking on sides of feet**

To build up your arches, walk on your toes, on your heels, or on the outside of your feet. Do this only as long as it feels comfortable.

Remember, you should never do anything that is too much of a strain or causes discomfort. The simplest exercise to strengthen arches is to walk barefoot on an uneven surface.

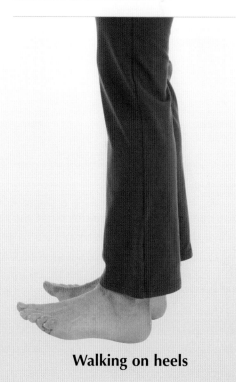

**Walking on heels**

# Well-positioned shoulders

The shoulder girdle is a complex structure, and one important component of it is the shoulder blades, which should lie flat against the back. Quite often, shoulder blades protrude away from the back; this is most often caused by a combination of strong/tight muscles at the front of the shoulders and weaker muscles at the shoulder blades. Correct Tai Chi practice should help to balance the muscles and flatten the shoulder blades.

Try the exercise below, rotating your arm in the shoulder socket and checking that your shoulder blades do not move during the process.

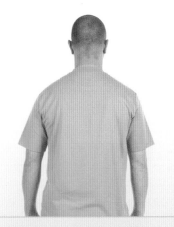 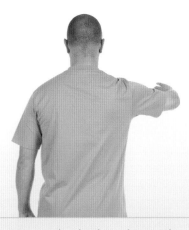 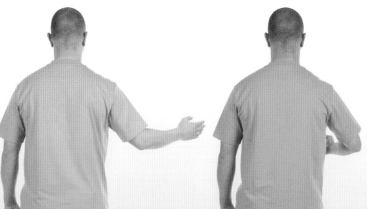

**1** Stand in the Basic Posture as explained on page 17.

**2** Put your hand in front of you as if touching a beach ball.

**3** Slowly move your hand in an arc to the side of the ball, then down, keeping your palm in contact with the ball.

**4** Slowly move your hand inside across your body with the elbow fixed.

**5** Move your hand back to the starting position and begin again.

You can check your shoulder blade movement (or lack thereof) during the exercise by putting your free hand on the lower tip of your shoulder blade. Alternatively, have someone else put their hand on the tip of your shoulder blade and tell you what they feel. If there is more than a small movement, practice these moves slowly while trying to keep the shoulder blade fixed until you become familiar with the sensation of a still shoulder blade.

## BAD POSTURAL HABITS

Most of us have minor postural problems that have accumulated through bad habits and poor use of our bodies. These problems will improve with correct practice and get a lot better when this results in improved habits! However, everybody is different, and what is a minor problem for one can be an injury waiting to happen for someone else. So if you feel you have postural problems that concern you, see a qualified professional.

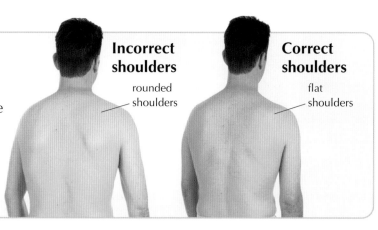

**Incorrect shoulders**
rounded shoulders

**Correct shoulders**
flat shoulders

# Standing practice in focus

Standing practice is the first step in training the stabilizing muscles that will help you to achieve effortless Tai Chi movement. This practice is called Zhan Zhuang, which means "standing like a pole." You should start doing standing practice from when you first start learning Tai Chi and continue for as long as you do Tai Chi. To progress well, you should practice Zhan Zhuang every day.

There are two positions for standing practice, positions 1 and 2. Practice only position 1 until you feel completely relaxed in it. This position is used mainly for relaxation and to correct posture. If you can, practice at about the same time each day.

When practicing Zhan Zhuang, you are mainly training your mind, so it's important to practice only when you have the energy to concentrate and pay attention to your body. If that means that you stand for only 5 or 10 seconds, that's fine—it's probably a good starting point.

Your ability to concentrate depends on your body awareness. If your awareness is low, your mind soon starts to wander. As you keep practicing Zhan Zhuang, your awareness will grow and you will naturally start to be able to concentrate for longer and therefore practice longer. When you concentrate, it's more enjoyable and you progress faster.

Gradually, extend your standing practice time to 5 or 10 minutes, and when it becomes effortless, you can practice standing for 20 minutes or even longer. Eventually, you will become accustomed to holding your body this way during everyday life and the standing practice will not be required.

## Zhan Zhuang—Position 1

Start in the Basic Posture (see page 17) and raise your arms in front of your body as if holding a balloon in front of your waist. Let your elbows hang down, and place the forearms in a horizontal position. Feel calm and balanced. Feel your body softening and any tension draining away. Keep your breathing soft and natural.

Pay attention to the quality of your standing. You will notice that your body is not quite still; there should be a constant small movement as your body adjusts your balance. Do not try to stop this movement (that would introduce tension); it is completely natural, and, in fact, it helps your stabilizing muscles to function better. As your awareness increases, the movements will gradually become smaller.

Later, when you have learned the Wuji Stance on page 40, you can further improve your posture in the Zhuan Zhuang position.

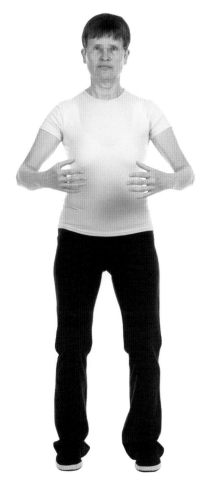

**Front view**

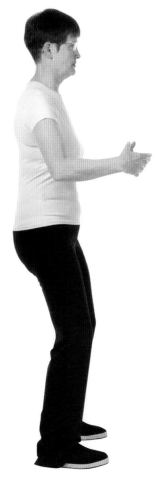

**Side view**

*(continued on next page)*

The second posture (position 2) of Zhan Zhuang is used to train the muscles that stabilize the body and to develop greater internal power. Only add this position to your standing practice when you have been practicing the first position long enough to feel relaxed.

As you continue practicing in position 2, you will eventually find your stance becoming more solid and you will have a feeling of fullness in your body. You will also find that you sleep better and any postural problems, such as backaches, will lessen.

Follow the advice given for position 1 for when to practice and for how long to practice. And remember, do standing practice only when you are able to concentrate fully.

## TAI CHI BREATHING

Because Tai Chi requires a lot of concentration, you may find you have a tendency to hold your breath while concentrating—so it is important to remember to breathe! Whether you are practicing static postures or moving exercises, always keep your breathing soft and natural, even and relaxed.

## Zhan Zhuang—Position 2

Start in the Basic Posture (see page 17), then move your feet farther apart and raise your arms in front of your body as if holding a balloon in front of your face. Feel as if your arms are floating effortlessly in space and as if you are trying to expand your whole body but there is some resistance outside that is preventing you.

Then, feel as if you are trying to squeeze your whole body inward but again some resistance is preventing you. Similarly, feel that you are trying to push the body up, down, forward, and back, and for each of these there is something preventing you.

Stay calm and balanced. Sense your body softening and any tension draining away.

Pay attention to the quality of your standing as you did for position 1 and remember to relax. Recognize that your body is constantly adjusting your balance and do not try to stop this movement. As your awareness increases, the movements will gradually become smaller.

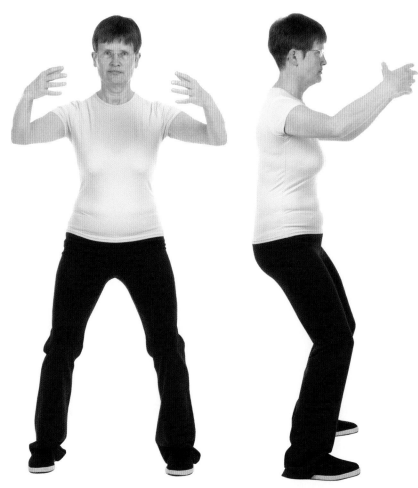

**Front view**          **Side view**

# 3 Warming Up

Whenever you practice Tai Chi, you should start by warming up. The following exercises will help you prepare your body for the slow, continuous Tai Chi movements, softening the muscles, loosening the joints, and improving coordination.

*A teacher leads you into the door; you walk your own way to your destination.*

—CHINESE PROVERB

Warming up for Tai Chi is more than just a warm-up. It is also aimed at improving the coordination of joints, so you need to pay careful attention to detail during each movement.

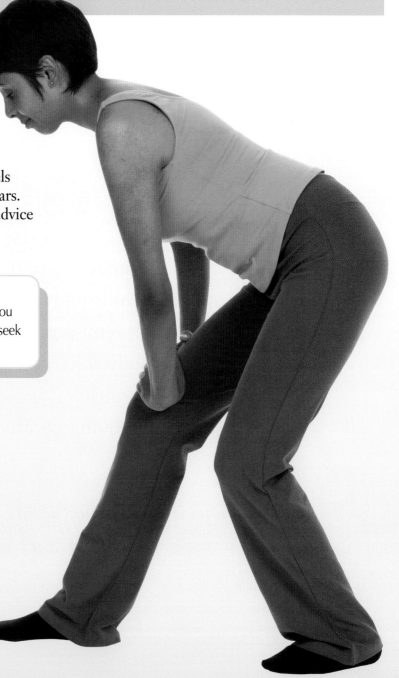

**W**arming up also softens the body, which makes it more sensitive. This is achieved by moving softly and slowly and relaxing the body and mind.

Although an amount or repetition is suggested, you can repeat each of the exercises in this chapter as many times as you like. Keep in mind that your eventual goal is to feel that you are involving your whole body in each exercise, moving the selected joints only as a focus of your awareness. This may be quite difficult to achieve at the beginning, so at first, practice the exercises until you feel comfortable and relaxed. Then gradually start noticing the subtle movements occurring in other parts of the body.

## Clicking joints during warm-ups

Some people might experience a "clicking" in the joints while moving, with no attendant pain or discomfort. This seems to happen most often in shoulders or hips, but it can occur in any of the joints. If it happens to you, do not ignore it; try to stretch the joint very slightly during the movement and move slowly and carefully through the position where you can feel the

"click." Try to find a joint position that feels comfortable and where the "click" disappears. If you can't, you should seek professional advice (see box).

### WARM-UP WARNING

If you experience any pain or discomfort when you are performing any Tai Chi exercise, you should seek professional advice about the cause.

# Swinging the arms side to side

The first thing you want to do when starting a warm-up is to relax the body. Rhythmically swinging the arms by moving the waist is an excellent way to do that.

Once you have learned this exercise, you can also use it as a practice to increase your body awareness. To do this, perform the exercise with your eyes closed and continue swinging 20–30 times. During this time, feel that you are exploring your body from the inside—sensing the space, observing physical sensations in your body, and feeling the movement of your joints.

If you keep practicing this way, the amount of detail you notice will continue to grow.

## FACE KNEES FORWARD

When performing this warm-up exercise, remember to keep your knees facing forward throughout the whole movement.

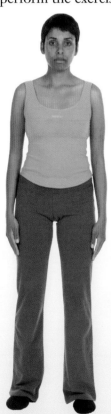 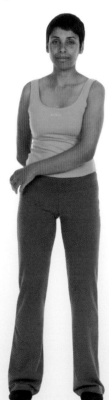 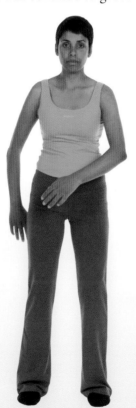 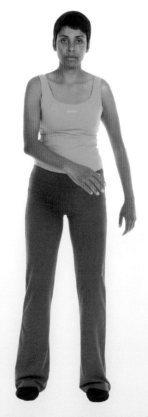 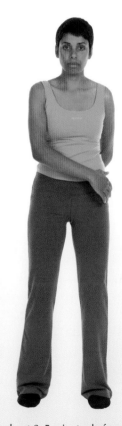

**Preparation:** Start in the Basic Posture (see page 17).
**Action:** Keeping your knees facing forward throughout the exercise, use only the rotation of your waist to swing your arms from side to side as shown above. The swinging movement should be soft and

relaxed. Let your shoulders feel the weight of your arms as they swing.

Once you are able to swing your arms freely, transfer a small amount of your weight from leg to leg as you swing—feel the weight of your body on each leg.

Continue swinging like this for about 2–5 minutes before moving on to the next arm exercise.

25

# Swinging the arms forward and back

In the previous exercise, you swung your arms around your body by rotating the waist. In this one, you swing your arms forward and back by bobbing up and down on your legs as you turn at the waist. As in the previous exercise, swing your arms in an easy rhythm and move your legs as if they are two springs being alternately compressed and released.

You should feel your arms being pulled down as you bend your knees and then feel them swing up using the momentum they gained on the way down. Feel the weight of the arms on your shoulders change from no weight when the hands are at their highest (about shoulder height) to several times their normal weight when the hands are at their lowest (next to your legs).

This exercise is excellent for improving the coordination of the waist with the legs and the arms.

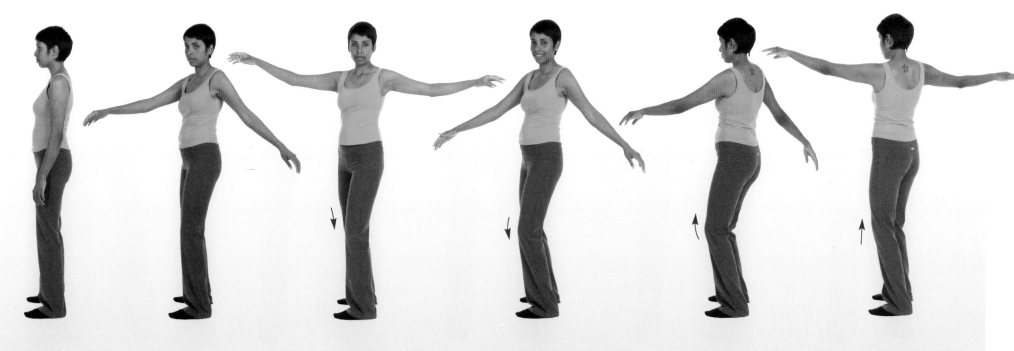

**Preparation:** Start in the Basic Posture with your feet shoulder-width apart.
**Action:** Swing your arms forward and back by rotating the waist and flexing the knees as shown above. When your arms start

moving down, bend your knees slightly and feel this movement pull your arms down. (Keep your knees facing forward throughout the exercise.) As your arms swing back up again, straighten your legs slightly (but not fully).

The swinging movement should be soft and relaxed. Feel the weight of your arms on your shoulders as the arms swing.
Swing your arms about 20–30 times before moving on to the next warm-up exercise.

# Circling the wrists

Now that you have relaxed your body with the arm-swinging exercises, you are ready to warm up the key joint areas.

Take your time with each exercise. First perform it softly as a warm-up routine, then gradually introduce a light stretch. Do not use force—a regular light stretch is all that is needed to make your joints stronger and more supple.

Your shoulders should stay relaxed throughout this exercise. When you are (softly) pushing one elbow up, make sure the shoulder on the same side remains settled down.

The elbows move up and down in a vertical direction (when one goes up, the other one goes down), with the one going up directly below the corresponding wrist. Check yourself in the mirror or ask someone to check your movements.

Perform the movements carefully and slowly at first. When you feel you can move without putting any strain on your wrists, you can speed up.

## POSITION SHOULDERS AND ELBOWS CORRECTLY

Make sure your shoulders remain relaxed and down. Your elbows should move up and down directly beneath your wrists.

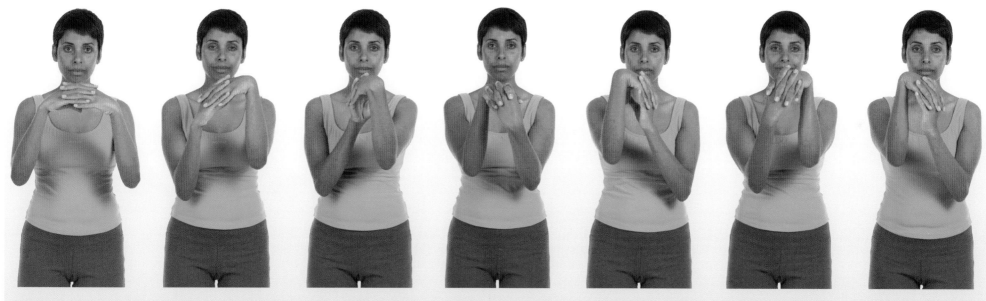

**Preparation:** Start in the Basic Posture with your feet shoulder-width apart, and relax into this position before you start. Raise your hands in front of you and interlock your fingers as shown above. Let your elbows sink down so that your forearms are parallel.

**Action:** Move your wrists forward and back, drawing a vertical, front-to-back circle with them, and at the same time move your elbows alternately up and down. Begin the movement by moving as softly as you can. As you relax into the movement, clasp your fingers firmly and keep a continuous pull between the arms as if you are trying to separate the hands. After a minute or so of rotating your wrists in one direction, rotate them in the opposite direction.

Rotate your wrists about 20 times in each direction.

# Rotating the elbows

This is an exercise to improve the flexibility of your elbows and the ability of your forearms to rotate. It is also an excellent exercise for improving the stability of your shoulders.

When practicing, avoid using the shoulders to help with the arm rotation. Keep the front of your shoulders open and the shoulder blades still.

If you can put one hand on your lower back and slide it up to touch the opposite shoulder blade (an excellent exercise in itself), you can check if your shoulder blades are moving as you perform this warm-up with one arm. If you cannot reach your shoulder blade, ask someone to check it for you while performing the exercise.

## KEEP HANDS AND SHOULDERS RELAXED

During this exercise hold your hands in loose, relaxed fists (see hand positions on page 43). Keep your shoulders relaxed and the shoulder blades still throughout this exercise.

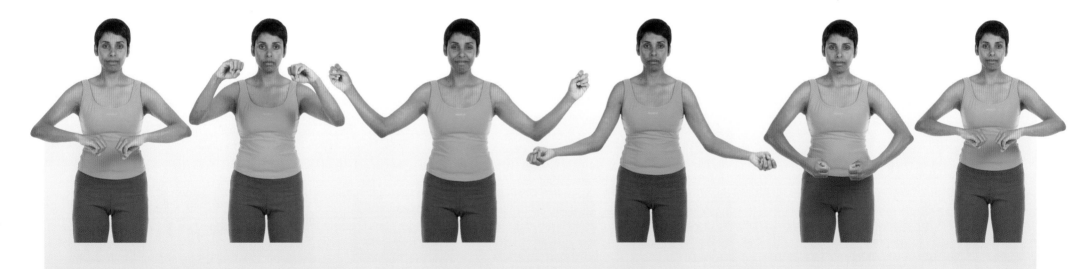

**Preparation:** Start in the Basic Posture. Raise your arms and bring your hands up in front of the chest, with the elbows sinking down but pointing away from the body.

**Action:** Circle your hands as shown above, moving them upward, slightly forward, out, and around back to the waist. At the same time, your elbows should also be making small circles. Rotate your forearms so that most of the time your palms face the center of each circle. Keep your knees soft, and gently move your body slightly up and down to match the up-down movement of your elbows.

Circle your arms about 20 times in one direction, then in the opposite direction before moving on to the next exercise.

28

# Rotating the shoulders

This is a great warm-up exercise for the shoulders and, in fact, the whole shoulder girdle and even the spine. During this exercise keep your shoulders down and the shoulder blades flat against your back, while sliding smoothly up and down.

After you become familiar with the movement of your arms and have your shoulder blades under control, move as suggested in the tip box on the right. Make sure you do not tense your shoulders to imitate the effort of pulling the imagined elastic bands. Keep your shoulders soft, but feel a slight resistance to your movement.

## USE THIS MENTAL IMAGE

During this exercise imagine that your elbows are joined to your ankles by weak elastic bands in order to sense that you are using your whole body (legs, spine, and arms) to circle your elbows.

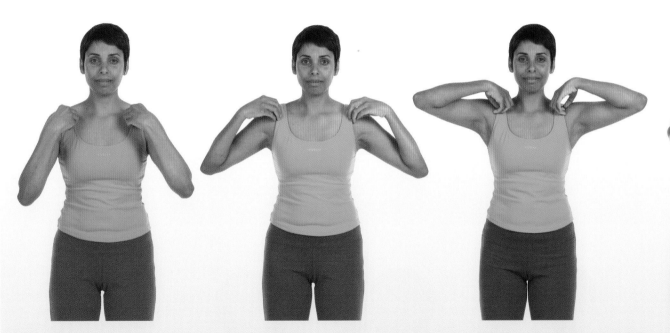
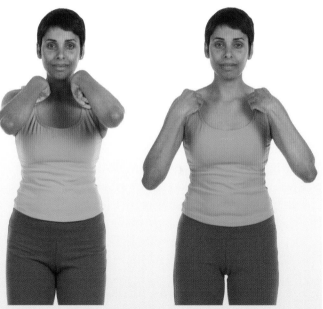

**Preparation:** Start in the Basic Posture. Then bring your fingertips together and place them on the front of your shoulders, letting your elbows sink down.
**Action:** Circle your elbows as shown above, bringing them up, forward, around, and back down to waist level. Make the circles as large as you can comfortably manage. Keep your knees soft and gently move your body slightly up and down to match the up-down movement of your elbows. When you lower your elbows (and bend your knees), feel your spine slightly bow as your chest and abdomen come toward each other a little. When you lift your elbows (and partially straighten your knees), feel your spine arch a little as your chest and abdomen separate slightly.

Circle your elbows about 20 times in one direction, then in the opposite direction before moving on to the next exercise.

# Mobilizing the neck and eyes

As long as your spine is in good condition, this is a safe exercise. Move slowly and softly, and pay close attention to the sensation in your neck. Your neck should move smoothly and quietly. Any discomfort, clicking, or other noises should be investigated by a professional.

Use your eyes to lead the movement of your head in these warm-ups. When looking up and lifting your chin, for example, first start looking up as if you are following something being lifted over your head. During all the movements, keep your head balanced and your neck soft.

"Look up and down" is a good exercise to use to increase body awareness. First perform the exercise as explained, then gradually make the movements smaller and smaller until you are not sure whether you are moving or whether you merely think you are moving. When you make these tiny movements that only you are aware of, observe how your head is balancing on your neck—which side of the neck you can feel more. You can do the exercise this way anywhere, and it is a great way to release tension in the neck, especially for the deskbound.

## START IN THE BASIC POSTURE

Before beginning the head and neck movements, relax into the Basic Posture and position your head correctly (see page 17). Feel your head floating up and your neck lengthening. Do not use any force when positioning the neck and head.

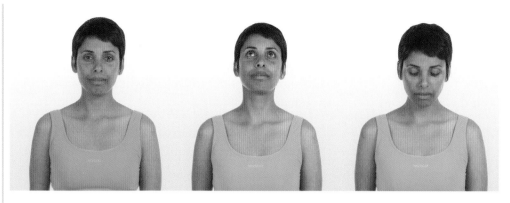

### Look up and down
**Preparation:** Start in the Basic Posture (see box).
**Action:** Look up as you slowly lift your chin up; do not allow the back of the head to hang down. Look down as you bring your chin back and slightly up, feeling the back of the neck lengthening.
   Move your head up and down like this about 10 times.

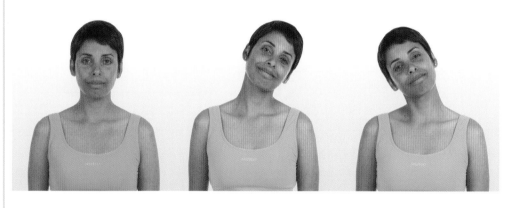

### Bend sideways
**Preparation:** Start in the Basic Posture (see box).
**Action:** Tilt your head to one side, lowering your ear toward the shoulder; do not move the head forward or back.
   Bend your head side to side like this about 10 times.

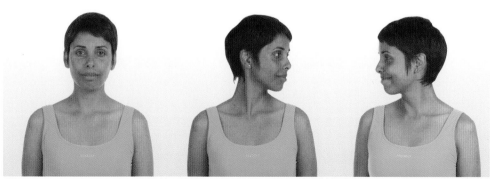

### Turn sideways
**Preparation:** Start in the Basic Posture (see box).
**Action:** Look to one side as if trying to look behind you, turning the head to follow the eyes. Look around as far as you can without straining. Then look to the other side.
   Turn side to side like this about 10 times.

# Opening the chest and upper back

This warm-up exercise is described in beats for clarity, but it is performed rhythmically and continuously in a flowing movement.

While doing the exercise, focus on the area between and under the shoulder blades. Notice this area open and close as you move your chest forward and back—one small move, one big move. The rib cage should feel soft and elastic. As your chest moves, sense the front and the back ribs separating and closing alternately. The more you mobilize the small intercostal muscles around the ribs, the better for your posture and breathing.

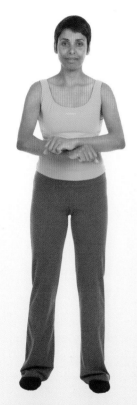

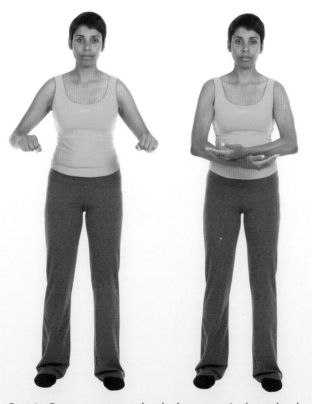

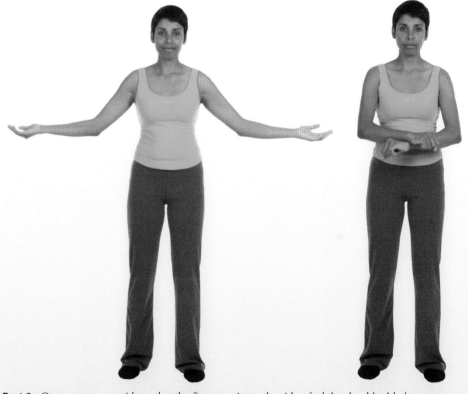

**Preparation:** Start in the Basic Posture. Cross your wrists in front of your waist, with the left arm on top, palms facing down, hands in loose fists.

**Beat 1:** Open your arms so that the forearms point forward and the chest moves slightly forward. Open your hands and turn them palms up as you cross your wrists again with the left arm on top while the chest moves back to its normal position.

**Beat 2:** Open your arms wide so that the fingers point to the sides; feel the shoulder blades come together and the chest open fully. As you close your arms, turn your hands palm down and close them into loose fists as you cross your hands again, but with your right wrist on top.

**Beats 3 and 4:** Repeat beats 1 and 2 with left and right reversed.

Repeat beats 1–4 about 10 times before moving on to the next warm-up exercise.

# Turning the lower back

The lower back is very important for your health and for Tai Chi development. The quality of movement in the lower back determines how well we can move from the center. The Tai Chi *Classics* say, "The waist is the commander of the whole body," and, "The source of the postures lies in the waist ... If you cannot get power, seek the defect in the legs and waist." In Chinese, the waist (*yao*) is the area of the lower back!

## MOVE SMOOTHLY

During the exercise, move smoothly and do not use force. Your spine is a column of small cylinders, each one moving a little more than the one below it.

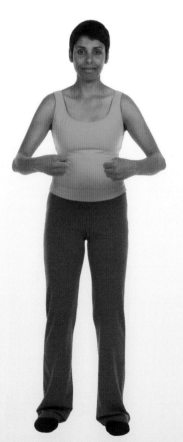 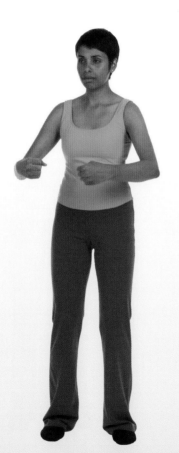 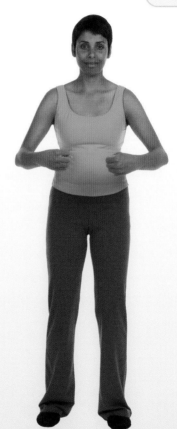 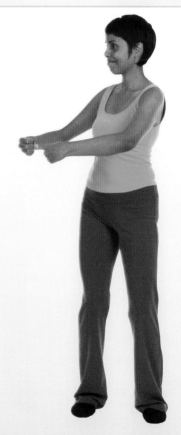

**Preparation:** Start in the Basic Posture. Keep your spine long and relaxed, especially the lower back. If necessary, bend your knees more to help the lower back relax. Hold your hands slightly apart in front of the waist, in loose vertical fists (thumb on top, little finger underneath).

**Action:** Keeping your knees facing forward throughout the exercise, rhythmically turn from your waist twice to one side, then twice to the other side alternately (only the turns to the right are shown above). On the first turn to each side, move from the hips so that the turn is small and the breastbone stays above the navel. On the second turn to each side, move from the waist so that the turn is larger and your breastbone now turns farther than the navel. Your head turns even farther, as if you are looking behind you. Move smoothly and softly. Feel the lower back widen and feel the elastic quality of the muscles in the lower and middle back. Repeat about 10–20 times.

# Circling the hips

Often our hips move either too much or too little. They are either too stiff or too weak. Most of the problems with the hips stem from the fact that we spend a lot of time sitting on chairs. This makes the deep supporting muscles of the abdomen weaker. Tai Chi stances are excellent for remedying this, but the process is gradual.

Hips connect the lower and upper body, and if the hips are stiff, it affects the whole body, especially the lower back. In this exercise, to free the hips and the lower back, focus on moving softly and on sensing the movement.

### MOVE HIPS CORRECTLY

When rotating your hips forward, be sure to move the hips, not the waist, and keep the lower back relaxed. When moving sideways, do not push the hip past your foot.

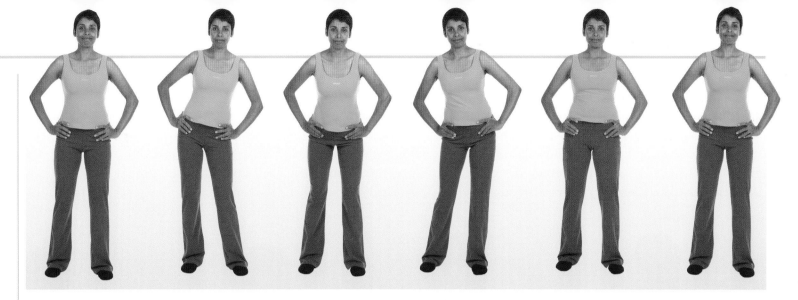

**Preparation:** Start in the Basic Posture with your feet shoulder-width apart. Place your hands on your hips. (This exercise is shown above face-forward and below as a side view, so that you can see both the sideways and the backward/forward movements clearly.)

**Action:** Keeping your knees slightly bent, slowly rotate your hips in a small circle. First rotate your hips in one complete circle in one direction and then rotate them in a complete circle in the other direction. Move smoothly and do not use force.

Rotate your hips about 10 times, then move on to the next warm-up exercise.

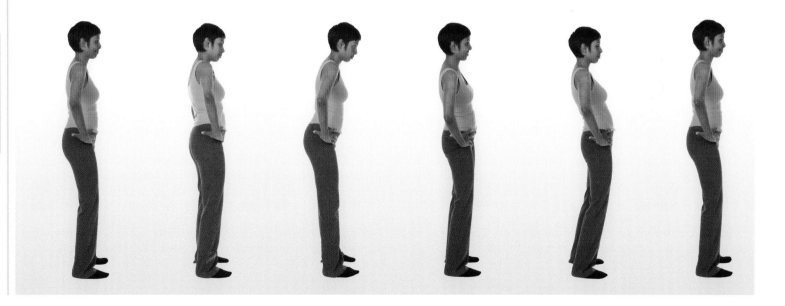

# Circling the knees

In terms of usage, the knee is a very simple joint—a hinge joint, just like the elbow. In terms of construction, however, the knee is probably the most complex joint in the body. It has to cope with the weight of the body, and it has to function well while under stress from all possible directions.

To keep your knees healthy, you need strong supporting muscles and good coordination of all the muscles around them. Tai Chi provides both, and this warm-up is the first step.

During the exercise, feel with your hands the tiny movements of the small muscles around the knee joints—these movements will strengthen and soften the knees.

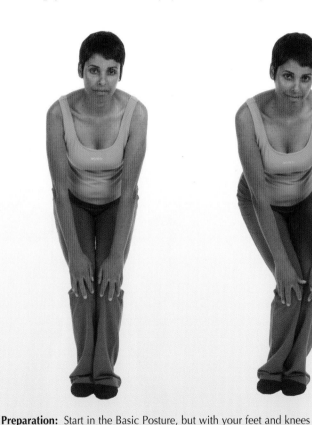
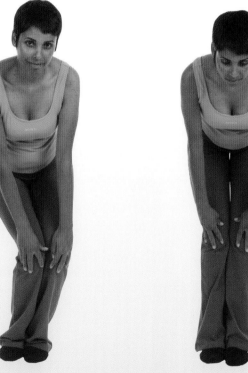
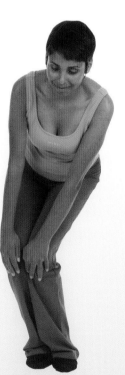
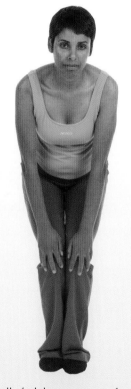
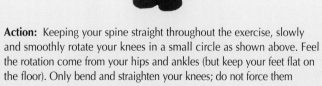

**Preparation:** Start in the Basic Posture, but with your feet and knees together. Bend your knees and place your hands lightly on your kneecaps.

**Action:** Keeping your spine straight throughout the exercise, slowly and smoothly rotate your knees in a small circle as shown above. Feel the rotation come from your hips and ankles (but keep your feet flat on the floor). Only bend and straighten your knees; do not force them sideways. Use your hands to continually feel the movement of your knees.

Repeat about 10–15 times in each direction before moving on to the next warm-up exercise.

# Circling the ankles and massaging toes

The ankle is another very complex joint. In fact, it is two joints together: one joint (the true ankle joint) is responsible for vertical motion, and the other (the subtalar joint) is responsible for sideways motion. Its intricate design is an engineering miracle, and this simple warm-up movement exercises it all.

Due to our modern lifestyle—wearing shoes on flat surfaces—our feet are constantly underused. There is a large part of the brain reserved for the feet, and we use only a small part of it—as the saying goes, "Use it or lose it." Tai Chi, fortunately, with its slow moves and single-leg stances, provides a challenge to our ankles—especially if practiced barefoot or in soft shoes, outside on grass, or other uneven surfaces.

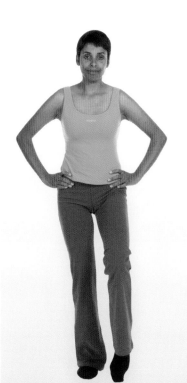
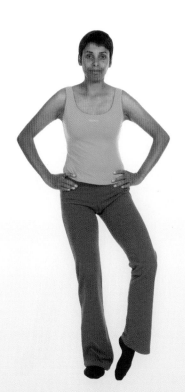
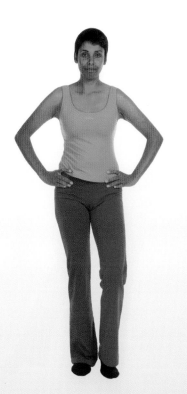
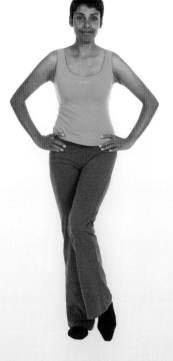
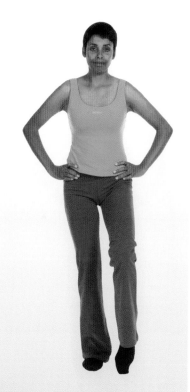

**Preparation:** Start in the Basic Posture. Then place your hands on your hips, transfer your weight to the right leg, and lift the left heel up, leaving the toes lightly touching the floor.

**Action:** Keeping your toes lightly touching the floor, slowly and smoothly rotate your ankle so that your heel moves in continuous circles in a counterclockwise direction as shown above. Next rotate the same heel again, but this time making circles in a clockwise direction. When circling, feel both the circling motion and the straightening and flexing of the ankle.

Rotate the left heel in one direction and then the other about 10–15 times. Repeat with the right heel.

# Circling the hips, knees, and ankles

alancing on one leg while circling the other leg is very tricky and will test your balance. Focus on the supporting leg and you will find that your balance improves immediately. With continued practice, the awareness of the joints will improve and with it the sense of control. The supporting ankle should feel strong and stable; do not allow it to wobble.

If you wobble during this exercise, find a spot on the floor about 6 feet (2 meters) ahead of you and fix your eyes on it—you may be surprised how focusing

on one spot improves your balance. As your balance improves, keep looking ahead, and later on you can look around freely.

Practice slowly until your ankle is stable and comfortable. Then increase your speed of circling and allow the circling motion into your supporting ankle; the ankle should feel steady with the weight in the foot circling around. This will further strengthen your ankle and improve your balance.

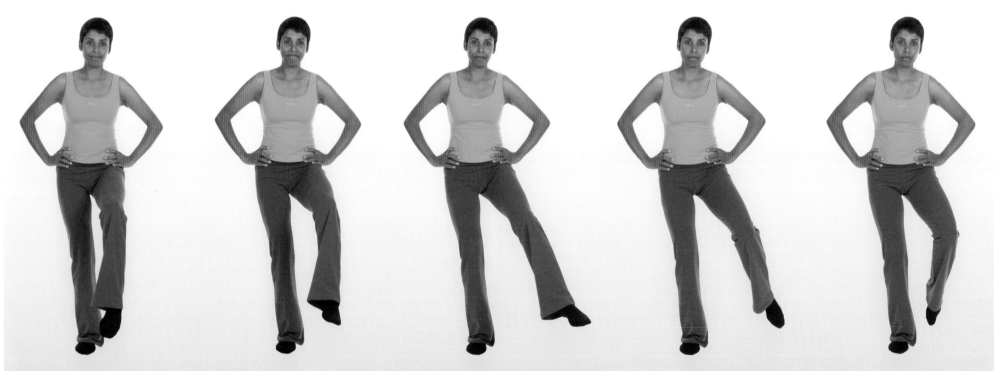

**Preparation:** Start in the Basic Posture. Then place your hands on your hips, transfer your weight to your right leg, and lift the left leg up with the knee bent and the lower leg hanging loosely down.

**Action:** With your toes, slowly and smoothly move in large horizontal circles in a counterclockwise direction as shown above. Keep your left hip, knee, and ankle soft and relaxed.

Then make circles in a clockwise direction. Perform about 20 circles in each direction.
Repeat with the right leg.

# Stretching and mobilizing the back

These are excellent exercises for keeping the spine young and healthy. The instructions for the Big Circle below describe how to move the hands and arms. Integrate these actions with the movement of the body. When the hands slide upward, slightly straighten your knees and lightly stretch your body up; when the hands move downward, slightly bend the knees and lightly compress your body. The spine should move in small waves as if the hands are sliding up the back of the spine, very lightly pushing it forward, and sliding down the front of the spine, very lightly pushing it back.

After familiarizing yourself with the Big Circle, use the same body movement in the Small Circle, only smaller and softer. Once you can practice the Small Circle movements with confidence, make them even smaller and softer, keeping the spine upright and feeling a wavelike motion in your back and body.

## Big Circle

**Preparation:** Start in the Basic Posture.
**Action:** Move your hands upward, with fingers hanging down, index fingers and thumbs touching the sides of the body, and elbows pointing sideways. When the hands reach the upper chest, rotate the elbows forward and down as you bring the hands together and slide them down with fingers pointing up and the "little-finger-edge" of your hands touching the body. When the hands reach the lower abdomen, move them outward to the sides and slide them up again to repeat the circle.

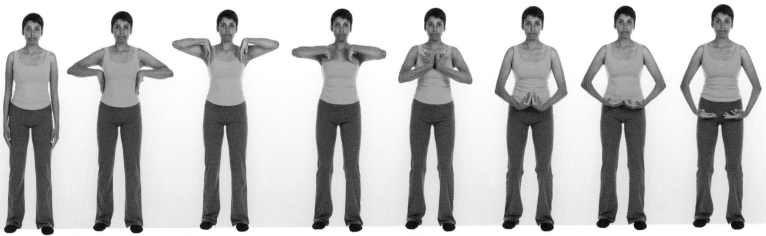

## Small Circle

**Preparation:** Start in the Basic Posture. Place your hands on the lower abdomen with elbows pointing sideways.
**Action:** Move your arms as for the Big Circle but keep your wrists at about the same level. Move your elbows in circles and rotate your hands at one spot. When your elbows move forward, feel your upper back bow; when the back of the wrists turn down, sink your body and feel your pelvis tilt back as the lower back bows. When your elbows move back, your spine straightens.

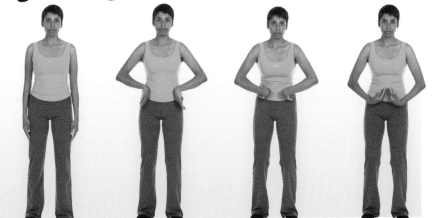

### KEEP IT SLOW

Keep all movements in these exercises integrated and slow. As you get used to the movements, you can move faster. Do not use any force.

# Stretching the calves and hamstrings

These warm-up exercises are designed to stretch and soften the calves and hamstrings—areas that can contain tension. Remember to do the exercises slowly and gently.

When you are softly bouncing the knee up and down to stretch your hamstrings, let the leg spring back naturally. If you feel the stretch in the back of the knee, bend the front leg more.

> **YOU SHOULD FEEL NO PAIN**
> Use very little force—you should feel a stretch but no pain.

## Calves

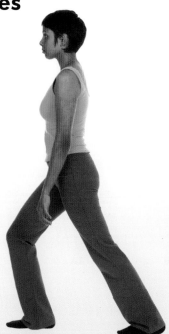 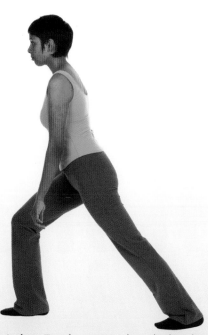

**Preparation:** Relax into the Basic Posture with the legs shoulder-width apart, then bend one leg and step straight forward with the other leg as shown above.

**Action:** Transfer your weight to the front leg and lean your body forward, feeling the calf of your back leg stretching. Experiment with the combination of the body leaning and the back leg straightening to produce the stretch. Move the front knee forward and back only. Do not let the knee go in front of the toes.
Repeat the stretch on the other side.

## Hamstrings

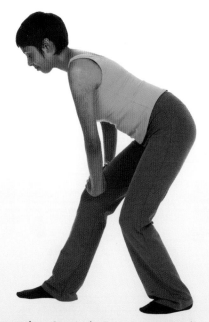 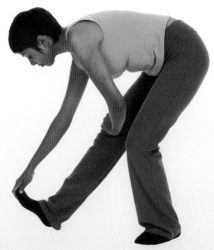

**Preparation:** Start in the Basic Posture. Bend your knees, put all your weight on one leg, and place the other leg 1 ft. (30 cm) in front, with the knee slightly bent. Keeping your spine straight, bend your body forward until you feel a light stretch in the hamstrings of the front leg. Place your hands on the front knee.
**Action:** Lightly and rhythmically press down and release your front knee by moving your

body; there should be a feeling of springiness in the leg as you softly bounce the knee up and down. After about 20–30 bounces, lift your front toes and hold them with one hand, then repeat the same action, this time adding a light pull on the toes when you press the knee down. If you cannot reach your toes, perform only the first part of this exercise.
Repeat the stretch on the other side.

# 4 Tai Chi Basics

In this chapter, you will learn the basic Tai Chi stances, hand positions, and Stepping. At this stage, spend just enough time with each of these basic elements for your body to relax into them. Perfecting them will come with practice later.

*When you practice Tai Chi, you should stand with your posture balanced like a scale.*

—FROM THE TAI CHI *Classics*

# LEARNING THE BASIC ELEMENTS

Before learning the sequence of Tai Chi postures and movements that make up the Form—a classic series of movements performed like a slow dance—you need to master the basics.

**WUJI GIVES BIRTH TO TAI CHI**
The Wuji Stance is used before performing the Tai Chi Form in order to center oneself. This is in accordance with the saying that "Wuji gives birth to Tai Chi."

Once you are familiar with these basic elements, you will find it much easier to remember the sequence of the Form later. Take your time and review the Tai Chi guidelines and tips on page 9 before you begin.

## Wuji Stance

The first stance you should try out is the Wuji Stance. The position for this stance is the same as the Basic Posture (see page 17). But to use the Basic Posture as the Wuji Stance, you must focus on achieving a perfect balance—both of the body and the mind. Treat this as an ongoing project and do not expect quick results. The better you balance, the less effort you will need to exert and the lighter your body will feel.

Eventually, with enough practice of the Wuji Stance, you will reach a state when your body feels as if it is totally empty or as if it is disappearing. This state of emptiness gives the stance its name—Wuji means "extreme emptiness."

To decide how much time to spend on this stance at this stage, see the guidelines on page 9.

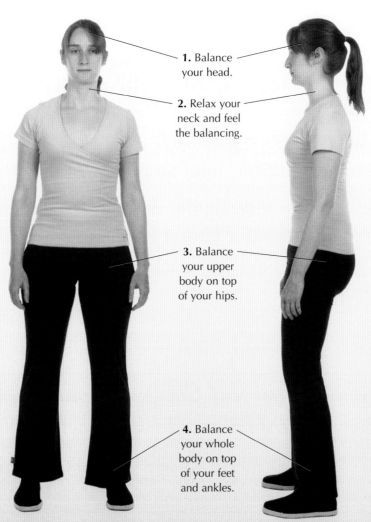

1. Balance your head.

2. Relax your neck and feel the balancing.

3. Balance your upper body on top of your hips.

4. Balance your whole body on top of your feet and ankles.

### Wuji Stance

Assume the Basic Posture on page 17. Then start the Wuji Stance by balancing your head. Relax your neck and feel it balancing.

Next, balance your upper body on top of your hips. Imagine your spine is a stick and use your pelvis as a hand to support the stick and balance your head on top of it.

Then balance your whole body on top of your feet and ankles. Feel your weight move between your heels and toes as you balance your body.

As your body awareness increases, the balancing movements will become gradually smaller and your body more quiet. At the same time, start subdividing your body into smaller segments. Eventually, it should feel as if you can balance through each individual vertebra.

# Bow, Cat, and Horse Stances

Here are the basic Tai Chi stances. In each of these stances, try to re-create the upper-body sensation that you experienced in the Basic Posture, especially the feeling of balance and relaxation. This will help to make them feel more natural. Try to become familiar with the way your body feels in these stances.

Hold each stance below for about five breaths (approximately 35 seconds). Feel your balance. Notice your weight sinking down and your hips, knees, and ankles relaxing.

There's no need to spend too much time on these stances—follow the guidelines on page 9.

## START IN THE BASIC POSTURE

Start all the stances on this page in the Basic Posture explained on page 17.

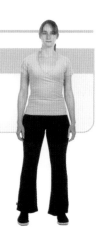

## Bow Stance

Start in the Basic Posture. Turn one of your legs out at an angle of about 45 degrees (pivoting at the hip joint), then take a step straight forward (so that your feet remain shoulder-width apart as seen from the front).

Transfer about two thirds of your weight to the front foot. Point both knees in the same direction as the feet. Make sure your front knee does not go over the toes and your lower back does not arch.

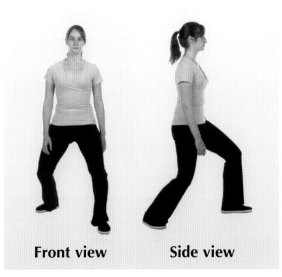

**Front view**     **Side view**

## Cat Stance

Start in the Basic Posture. Turn one of your legs out at an angle of about 45 degrees (pivoting at the hip joint). Lift the other knee up and forward so that your foot comes off the floor, then lower the leg down until the tip of your relaxed foot touches the floor. Do not put any weight on your front foot.

Point both knees in the same direction as the feet. Keep your hips level.

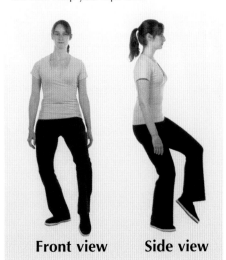

**Front view**     **Side view**

## Basic Horse Stance

Start in the Basic Posture. Step to the side so that the feet are about twice shoulder-width apart. Turn the feet slightly out. The knees should point in the same direction as the feet. Keep your hips level, and balance your weight equally on each foot.

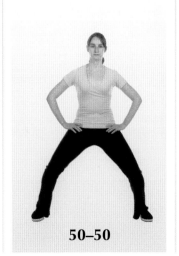

**50–50**

## Horse Stance 60–40

Start with the Basic Horse Stance, then transfer your weight to the left side so that your weight distribution is about 60–40 (60 percent on the left leg and 40 percent on the right leg).

Point the knees in the same direction as the feet. Keep your hips level.

Repeat, transferring your weight to the right side.

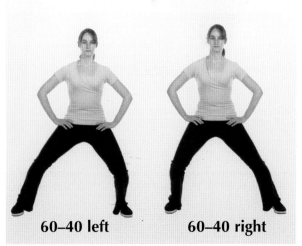

**60–40 left**     **60–40 right**

# Getting into the Basic Stance

Having learned a few stances, you now need to know how to move into the Basic Stance. This exercise will help you gain greater body awareness, which is essential in Tai Chi. It also happens to be exactly how you will start your Tai Chi Form later.

After learning the sideways step below, start paying attention to how your body feels while performing the movement. Keep repeating it for a while; move slowly and deliberately and pay attention to your balance all the time. Experiment with how it feels when you make small alterations to the movement, perhaps by starting with step 5 and reversing the movements.

As you practice, slowly and gradually you will become aware of more subtle sensations, more areas of your body. As your awareness increases, your movement will become more natural. For example, with practice you will know how far to sink in step 2 so that in step 4 the right knee doesn't straighten or remain too bent.

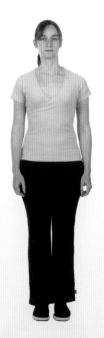 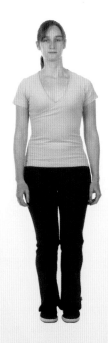 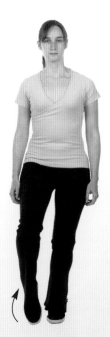 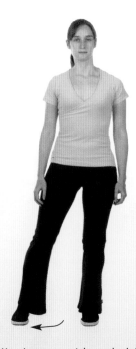 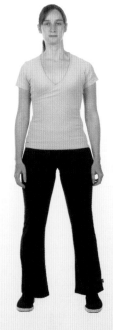

**1** Start in the Basic Posture, but with the feet together. Relax into this position.

**2** Keeping well-balanced and relaxed, bend both knees a little to sink slightly down as shown above.

**3** Keeping the left knee flexed, slowly sink all your weight onto the left leg and lift the right heel, leaving the toes on the floor.

**4** Keeping your weight on the left leg, step the right leg one shoulder-width to the right and lower your heel. Keep your right knee slightly flexed.

**5** Without changing the bend in the right knee, push off the left leg until your weight is evenly distributed between the two feet. Sink and relax.

# Tai Chi hand positions

The three main hand positions in Tai Chi are Fist, Beak, and Palm. According to the Tai Chi *Classics*, the internal energy is "rooted in the feet, generated in the legs, directed by the waist, and expressed in the hands and fingers."

For the correct expression, the hands must be relaxed and comfortable—but not limp. With practice, you will eventually feel as if all the joints in the hand are slightly inflated from within.

Your hand, regardless of whether it is in the Fist, Beak, or Palm position, should have a "hollow" center. This refers to a feeling in the hand that the palm is carefully wrapped around something soft and fragile. The back of the hand should feel stretched.

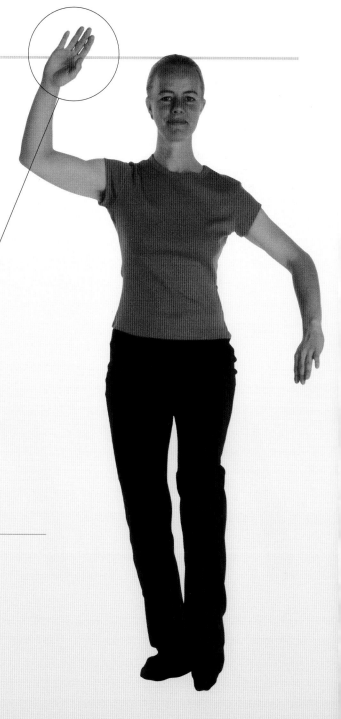

## Fist—solid

- Relaxed
- Back of the wrist straight

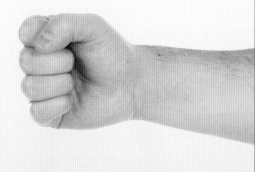

**Side view**

## Beak—focused

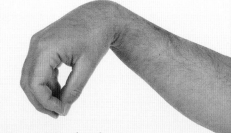

- Fingers joined at the tips
- Wrist arched
- Focus at the fingertips

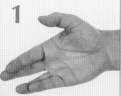

To position fingers correctly, first overlap fingers as shown above (1). Then keeping them in this position, move the fingertips and thumb together (2).

## Palm—soft

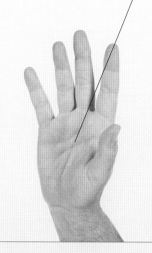

- Fingers rooted in the palm
- Wrist straight or seated
- Whole hand relaxed

# Whole-body Tai Chi movement

When you move in Tai Chi, you want every part of your body to contribute. Before moving on to learn basic Stepping, take a close look at whole-body movement—this will help you understand the basics of Tai Chi movements.

The Tai Chi *Classics* say, "When one part of the body moves, there is no part that does not move. When one part of the body is still, there is no part that is not still." In other words, either everything moves or nothing moves. This describes the all-pervasive movement that is a prerequisite for whole-body power.

The basis for this whole-body movement is, as explained in Chapter 2, relaxation and the use of postural muscles (the muscles that balance the body). When you lift an arm, this alters the position of your center of gravity, and your body rebalances along its entire length. This happens naturally if there is no stiffness or tension in any areas of the body.

To learn to move like this, you have to move slowly while paying attention to your balance and eliminating any tension. It helps if you treat Tai Chi movement as a "flow" of postures and become aware of the underlying postures. Try the arm movements below to investigate whole-body movement.

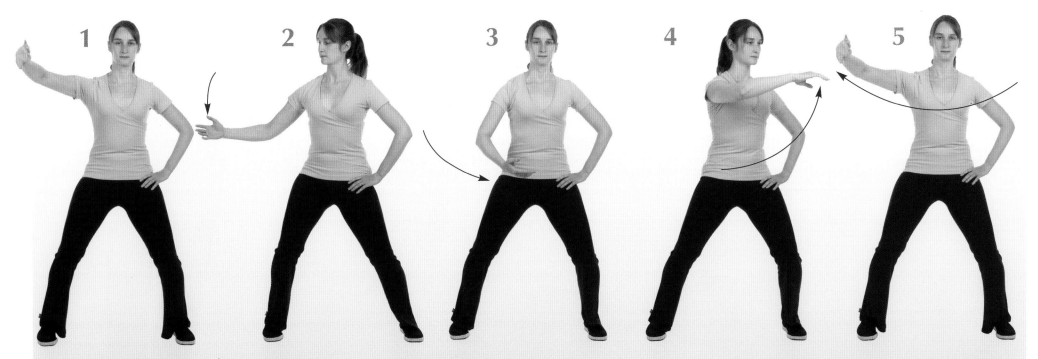

1  2  3  4  5

Standing relaxed in the Basic Stance, try slowly circling the right arm as shown above and see whether you can engage the whole body in the process. (For the time being, ignore the left arm, which is "parked.")

Notice how the arm twists slightly along its length, as do the legs and the upper body. Make the twisting an even and smooth, single twisting action through the whole body.

Experiment for a while with the way the spiral in the limbs and the body interact with each other. Does the twisting start in the legs, body, or arms? Is the leg connected with the same or the opposite arm? At this stage there are no right or wrong answers to these questions, because you are simply exploring how your body moves and reacts to the movement.

Later you will use this whole-body twisting action in Silk-Reeling motion and Silk-Reeling strength as explained on pages 53–66.

# Stepping (like a cat)

ow that you have seen basic Tai Chi stances, hand positions, and whole-body movement, you are ready to start Tai Chi Stepping. The method of Stepping is designed to facilitate balance throughout, help to develop a solid base, and enable an instant change of direction at any point.

Before trying Stepping forward, backward, sideways, or diagonally, practice the exercise below. It explains how you move your legs through space when performing Stepping in any direction. The mental image suggestion will help you perfect the technique.

When you get comfortable with "carrying" your foot simply forward and backward, start moving it in a horizontal circle—three times one way, three times the other way. As you get better, increase the number of circles to five and later to 10.

## Rolling a pencil

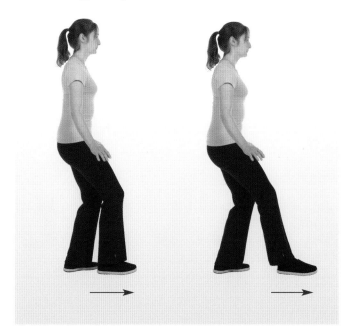

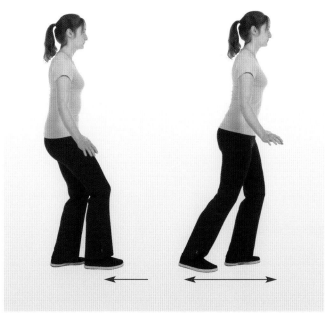

1 Start in the Basic Posture. Spread your arms to the side to help you balance. Transfer your weight to the left leg, and lift your right knee to lift the right foot off the floor, leaving just a small gap underneath it. Pretend there is a pencil on the floor and move your foot forward, as if you are very slowly rolling the pencil forward.

2 Then move your foot backward as if slowly rolling the pencil backward. Perform the movement forward and back three times on each side, always looking straight ahead, not at the floor. Keep your foot parallel to the floor throughout the whole movement (do not raise the toes when the foot is in front, or the heel when it is in the back).

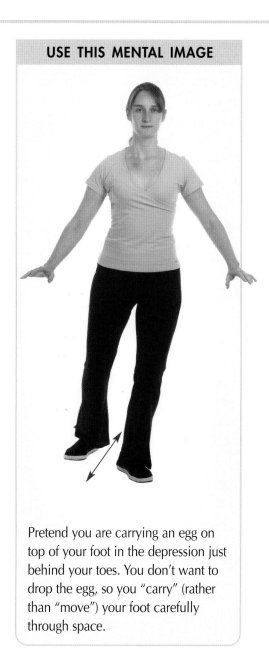

# Stepping forward

**T**ai Chi Stepping differs from the way you step during normal walking in two respects: the way your legs move through space and the way your weight is transferred.

In normal walking you swing your legs forward. In Tai Chi Stepping you move your legs by "carrying" them as you practiced in the "Rolling a pencil" exercise on page 45.

In normal walking you move your weight forward continuously, which makes you "fall" onto the moving leg as it touches the floor. In Tai Chi Stepping, you do not move the weight of your body forward when a leg moves through space. That means that all your weight is transferred off the leg that is being lifted and no weight is shifted forward toward the moving leg before the foot touches the ground.

Practice Stepping forward as explained below. Take into account the tips in the box, move slowly, and keep the movement flowing as you step forward.

"Rolling a pencil" exercise on page 45

## FOLLOW THESE TIPS

- Try keeping your hips the same height; do not move up and down.

- Look ahead, not down—feel your head suspended from above.

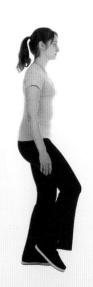 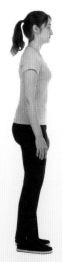 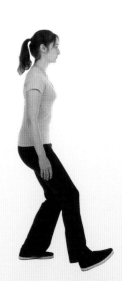 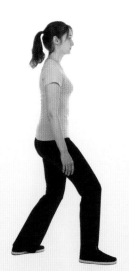 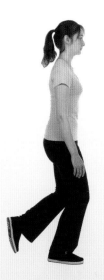 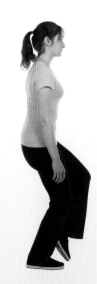 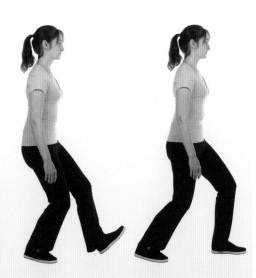

**1** Start in the Basic Posture, but with your feet together. Relax into this position before starting.

**2** As you lift the right heel off the floor (leaving the toes just touching the floor), sink all your weight onto the left leg.

**3** Lift your right knee so that your toes come off the floor, and "carry" your right foot forward. Before your knee fully straightens, lower the foot until the heel touches the floor.

**4** As you transfer your weight forward, lower the toes to the floor. Continue to move the front knee steadily in the same direction as the front foot is pointing.

**5** As you sink all your weight onto the front foot, slowly lift the rear heel, leaving the toes touching the floor.

**6** Lift the toes and move the rear foot slowly forward until next to the front foot, placing only the toes on the floor.

**7** Carry the left foot forward and then the right, and continue stepping forward with one foot after the next.

Review the tips on the next page to try to improve your Stepping practice.

# Stepping feet in focus

When you lift a leg during the Stepping practice, start by lifting your knee with your foot just hanging relaxed below the knee.

Move the foot forward at a slight angle toward the outside. When you place the heel on the floor, keep looking ahead and feel the floor as if you are not certain about the surface.

When you begin practicing Stepping forward, touch the toe of your back foot to the floor as it reaches the front foot. Gradually, with practice, your balance and confidence will improve so that you can bring your foot forward without the toes touching the floor.

*According to the Tai Chi Classics, the internal energy is "rooted in the feet, generated in the legs."*

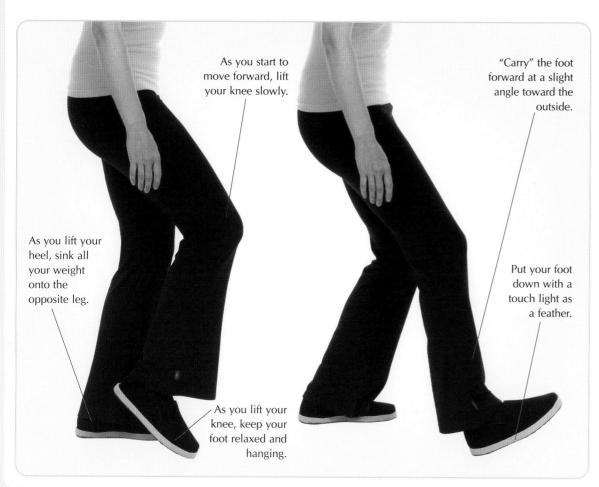

As you start to move forward, lift your knee slowly.

As you lift your heel, sink all your weight onto the opposite leg.

As you lift your knee, keep your foot relaxed and hanging.

"Carry" the foot forward at a slight angle toward the outside.

Put your foot down with a touch light as a feather.

## Shifting weight

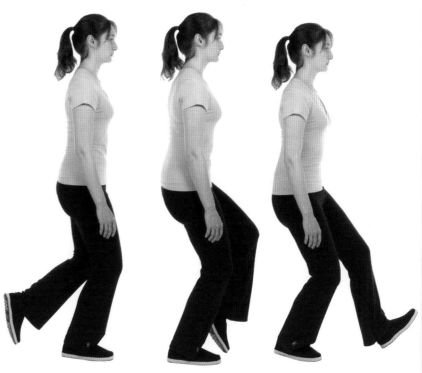

Once you are confident with your Stepping, bring the back foot forward in a single, slow, flowing movement without the toes touching the floor and without pausing.

Do not shift your weight while your foot is off the ground. Shift your weight only when both feet are on the floor.

# Stepping backward

As far as movement of the body and legs is concerned, Stepping backward is the exact reverse of Stepping forward.

We do not usually make a habit of walking backward, but when we try to do so, it is more like Tai Chi Stepping than when we walk forward. Usually the back leg touches the floor before we start transferring body weight backward, and we also tend to "carry" the leg back more than when we walk forward.

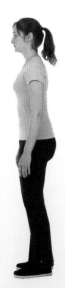 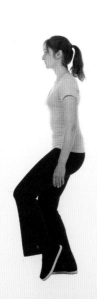 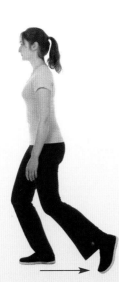 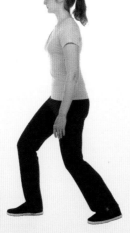 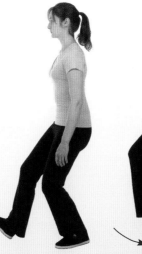 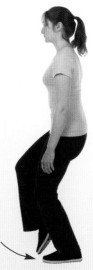 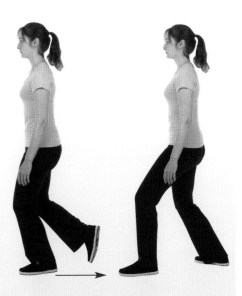

1 Start in the Basic Posture, but with your feet together. Relax into this position before starting.

2 As you lift the left heel off the floor (leaving the toes just touching the floor), sink all your weight onto the right leg.

3 Lift your knee so that your toes come off the floor, and slowly "carry" your left foot backward and out at a slight angle.

4 Place the toes on the floor, then transfer your weight backward as you lower the heel.

5 As you sink all your weight onto the back foot, lift the toes of the front foot.

6 Lift your heel off the floor, and move the front foot backward next to the back foot, placing only the toes on the floor.

7 Carry on Stepping slowly backward in this way. As your Stepping improves, begin moving the front foot backward without the toes touching the floor and without pausing.

# Stepping diagonally

While Stepping forward and back is often used in a sequence of Tai Chi steps, diagonal Stepping is usually used to move in and out of stances. The main difference between diagonal and other Stepping is that in diagonal Stepping, the leg moving forward remains in contact with the floor. But there should still be no weight on the moving foot; you should "carry" it forward, touching the floor only lightly.

Stepping diagonally, your path follows a zigzag line. Keep your eyes looking forward and move slowly and deliberately.

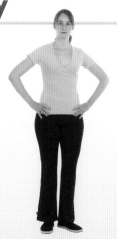

**1** Start in the Basic Posture but with the feet together. Place hands on hips and turn the left foot out at a 45-degree angle.

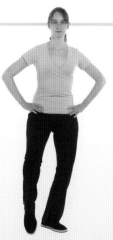

**2** As you lift the right heel off the floor (leaving the toes just touching the floor), sink all your weight onto the left foot.

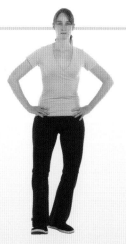

**3** Lift your right knee so that your toes come off the floor, and as you lift the toes, place your heel where your toes were.

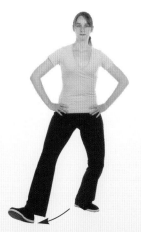

**4** Slowly slide your right foot diagonally forward with your foot still pointing forward and the heel lightly skimming the floor. At the same time, bend your supporting leg farther so that you can make a full step without having to transfer any weight.

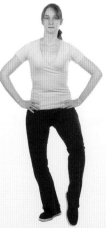

**5** Lower the toes down as you transfer your weight forward, moving the front knee steadily in the same direction the foot is pointing.

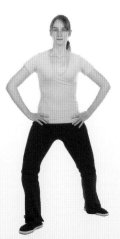
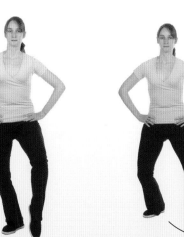

**6** As you sink all your weight onto the front foot, slowly lift the rear heel, leaving the toes touching the floor. Lift the toes and move the rear foot slowly next to the front foot, placing only the toes on the floor. Again lift your knee so that your toes come off the floor, and carry on Stepping.

## TURN THE HIPS

As you slowly step diagonally forward in step 4, stop before your front knee fully straightens. Turn your hips toward the front foot—use this action to turn the front leg out so that the leg and the foot are in line.

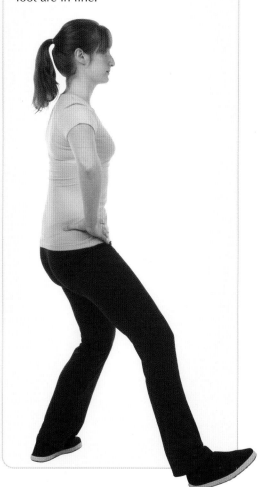

# Stepping sideways

When you step sideways in the Form, you always look in the direction you are traveling before you perform the step. In this practice, however, you should look forward. This is to help you practice feeling the position of your leg rather than actually seeing where it is.

Repeat this movement until you are confident in predicting when your foot will touch the ground. Try this in the other Stepping practices, too.

Once you can step sideways with confidence, lift your toes and heels only slightly, leaving your feet nearly horizontal.

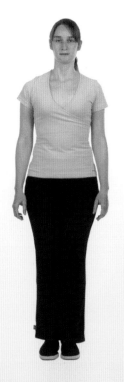 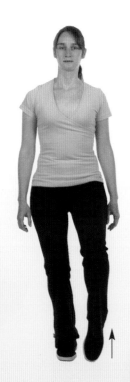 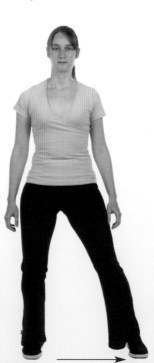 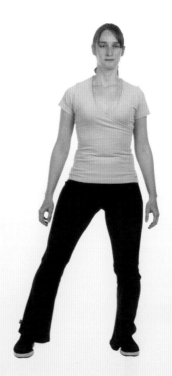 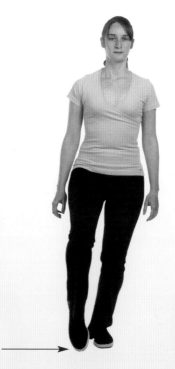 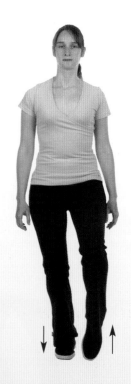

**1** Start in the Basic Posture but with the feet together. Relax into the position. (Look ahead during the whole exercise.)

**2** As you lift the left heel off the floor (leaving the toes just touching the floor), sink all your weight onto the right leg.

**3** As you lift your toes, slowly "carry" the left foot sideways. Then lower your heel so that it touches the floor. Lower the toes to the floor, making sure that the feet are parallel.

**4** Transfer your weight to the left leg.

**5** Slowly lift the right heel and slowly move the right foot next to the left one, placing only the toes on the floor.

**6** Lower the right heel down as you sink your weight onto the right leg while lifting the left heel. Carry on Stepping to the left. After several steps, reverse the direction and step toward the right.

50

# Stepping forward—arm movements only

Before combining arm movements with your Stepping, practice the arm movements while standing in the same place as explained below. The arms are moving in opposite direction to each other throughout the movement. Coordinate the waist and arm movement.

## Front view

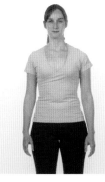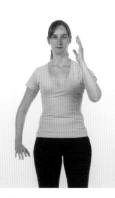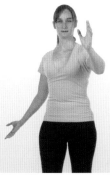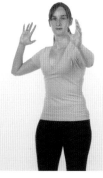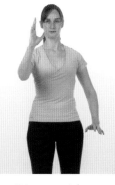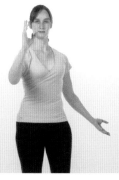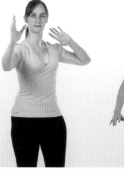

**1** Start in the Basic Posture but with the feet together.

**2** Lift the left arm and move the hand to about 1 ft. (30 cm) in front of the shoulder, with the edge of the palm facing forward and fingers pointing up. At the same time, press the heel of the right hand back so that the fingers lift up and point forward.

**3** Slowly rotate the waist to the right, while the right shoulder rotates outward, opening the front of the shoulder. Rotate the right arm clockwise until the palm faces to the right. At the same time, push the left arm forward, keeping the elbow bent.

**4** Start lifting the right arm back and up until it is about 1 ft. (30 cm) behind your right ear. At the same time, move the left hand forward and slightly down.

**5** Bring your right hand toward and past the right ear as you move your left hand down and then slightly back. At the same time, start turning your waist toward the front.

**6** Keep turning your waist as you push the right hand forward and the left hand down and back.

**7** Start lifting the left arm back and up until it is about 1 ft. (30 cm) behind your right ear. At the same time, move the right hand forward and slightly down.

**8** Bring your left hand toward and past the left ear as you move your right hand down and then slightly back. At the same time, start turning your waist back toward the front. Continue rotating the arms in this way.

## Side view—showing extension of arms

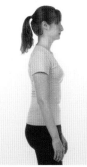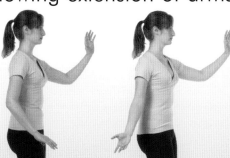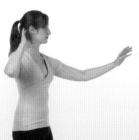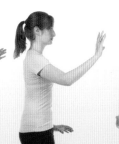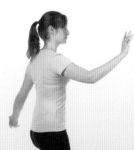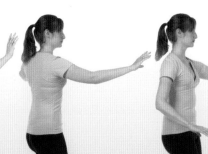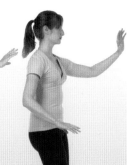

# Stepping forward—arms and legs together

Once you have mastered the arm movements for Stepping forward, you are ready to combine them with the leg movements. Be sure to keep looking ahead while Stepping. Coordinate the waist, arm, and leg movements. If you have difficulty doing this, practice the feet and arm movements separately again.

When you can step with confidence, do not put the toes of the rear foot on the floor as you bring it next to the front foot, but move both the leg and the arm forward in a slow, continuous, flowing movement.

Try to keep your hips at the same height, and do not move up and down.

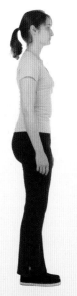 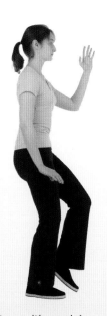 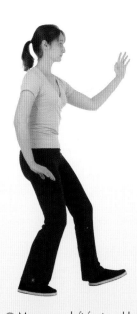 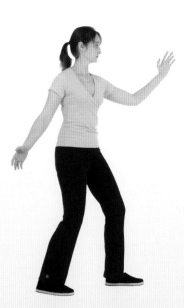 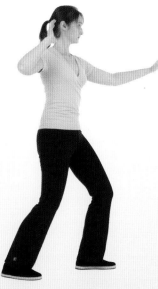 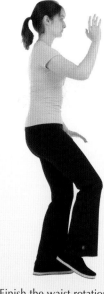

**1** Start in the Basic Posture but with the feet together.

**2** As you lift your left arm, with your left elbow above the left knee, lift your left heel off the floor.

**3** Move your left foot and hand forward at a slight angle, keeping the left elbow above the left knee. As the left hand moves forward, press the heel of the right hand slightly backward.

**4** As you rotate the waist to the right, transfer your weight halfway forward. At the same time, push the left hand forward and rotate the right hand backward.

**5** As you rotate the waist back toward the front, transfer your weight forward. At the same time, move the left hand slightly down and back, and the right one up and forward toward the ear.

**6** Finish the waist rotation by bringing the right foot next to the left, with the toes touching the floor. At the same time, bring the left hand back to just in front of the left leg, and the right hand past the ear to just in front of your right shoulder, with the edge of the palm facing forward.

You are now ready to step forward with your right leg.

**CHAPTER**

# 5 Silk Reeling

The smooth, soft, and continuous turning and twisting of Silk Reeling exercises involve the whole body. This spiraling of the body is the basis of all movement in Tai Chi. These flowing movements are a joy to learn and are the basis for the Form.

*Rotate the waist like a wheel.*

—FROM THE TAI CHI *Classics*

# ABOUT SILK REELING

Silk Reeling evenly stretches your whole body, exercises all your joints, and strengthens your muscles. Silk Reeling requires concentration, but it is a fundamental part of the Form, so practicing regularly will help you to learn more about your body and how you move.

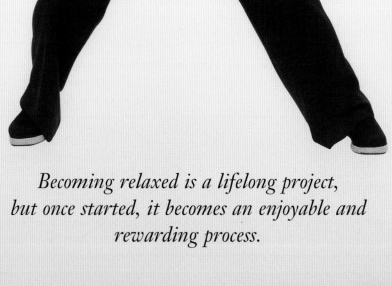

The turning and twisting movement of Silk Reeling strengthens the whole body because it engages every muscle. Apart from its use in martial art, the constant spiraling of the body is very beneficial for your health—it exercises your joints without strain while stretching every part of your body.

Silk Reeling exercises are said to promote the proper circulation of *chi* (internal energy).

## Relax the body

For the spiraling movement of Silk Reeling to travel freely through your body, you need to be relaxed. So before moving on to the preparation exercises on the following pages, make sure your body is not tense. If you feel any tension at all, use the warm-up exercises in Chapter 3 to help you relax. The exercises for shoulders, upper and lower back, hips, and spine ("Stretching and mobilizing the back") are especially good for relaxation. Then perform each of the Silk Reeling exercises slowly and attentively. They will also gradually relax and soften your body.

## Practice regularly

You should practice Silk Reeling exercises until they feel comfortable and natural. This will take some time; you should think in terms of months rather than days. Practice regularly and often before attempting the Form, and then, to improve your Silk Reeling, continue to practice while you are learning the Form.

*Becoming relaxed is a lifelong project, but once started, it becomes an enjoyable and rewarding process.*

# **Preparation**—moving the *dantian* left and right

Before starting to practice Silk Reeling, follow the preparation exercises on this and the following three pages. They introduce you to what the Chinese call the *dantian*—an essential concept in Tai Chi practice.

In Tai Chi, the *dantian* is the coordinating center of the body. Think of it as a ball lying within the lower abdomen that you can manipulate with your mind.

When you first start to learn Silk Reeling, you will be focusing on coordinating your arms, body, and legs. But once you have memorized the moves, you should gradually shift the emphasis toward feeling as if the *dantian* is leading and the body is following.

Start the Silk Reeling preparation exercises by moving the *dantian* left and right, shown below. Repeat each exercise about 10 times before moving on to the next preparation exercise.

## **Seated**

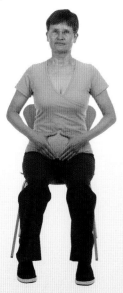 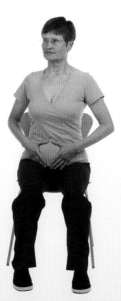 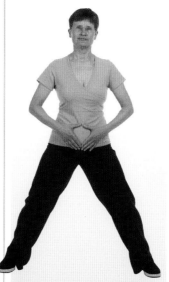

1 Sit on a chair with your feet shoulder-width apart and your heels beneath the knees. Place your hands on the lower abdomen, with the palms and fingers gently resting on the body and the thumbs pointing toward each other as shown above.

2 Twist your body slowly from side to side by moving your lower abdomen. First, feel as if your hands are moving a ball in your abdomen (later you should try to feel as if the ball—the *dantian*—is carrying your hands around). Make sure the movement is not coming from your waist or chest. The chest, waist, and the lower abdomen should move as one unit.

Repeat about 10 times. The movement is likely to be very small—perhaps hardly noticeable at first. As the body relaxes, the movement will become easier.

## **Standing**

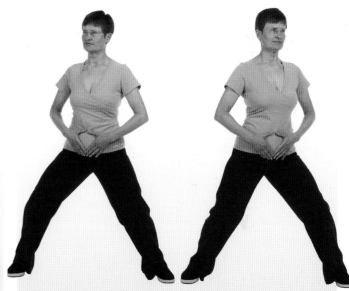

1 Stand in a wide stance that is comfortable, with your knees slightly bent and your hands on the lower abdomen, with the thumbs pointing toward each other and your little fingers on the groin as shown above.

2 Relaxing your hips so there is no resistance to movement, turn your body from side to side as in the seated exercise, but this time feel as if your *dantian* is pulling your hips around. Your knees should not move, and you should feel, with your little fingers, the groin closing and opening. The chest, waist, lower abdomen, and pelvis should move as one unit.

Repeat about 10 times. If you feel any sideways movement or sideways force in your knees, keep focusing on relaxing your hips.

# Preparation—rocking the *dantian* forward and back

**H**aving practiced moving the *dantian* left and right, you will now have an understanding of the position of the *dantian* in the body and a feeling for sideways rotation of the *dantian*. The exercise on this page will familiarize you with the forward-back movement of the *dantian*. Being seated will make it easier to feel the movement of your spine in the lower back (the lumbar region).

While learning the movements below, focus on the imaginary ball in your abdomen (the *dantian*) rocking forward and back.

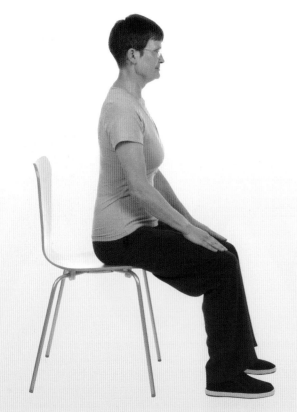

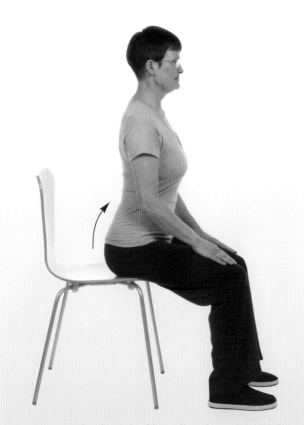

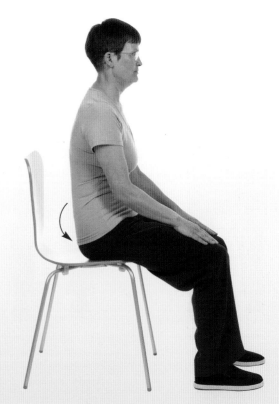

**1** Sit forward on a chair with your body upright, feet shoulder-width apart, and heels beneath your knees. Gently rest the palms of your hands on your knees, with fingers pointing forward.

**2** Keeping your head and shoulders still, rock your lower abdomen and lower back forward and back on the "sitting" or "sitz" bones (the lowest points of the pelvis). Feel as if you are rolling the

imaginary ball in the abdomen (the *dantian*) over the sitz bones. Move smoothly and slowly in a continuous motion. Repeat 10 times before moving on to the next exercise.

# Preparation—rotating the *dantian*

Rotating the *dantian* combines the seated exercise on page 55 and the rocking exercise on page 56. Move slowly and deliberately and make sure the movement is not coming from your waist or chest. The chest, waist, and the lower abdomen should move as one unit. Imagine that your *dantian* is moving like a ball tethered at its base.

Perform the exercise in both directions, rotating the *dantian* clockwise and counterclockwise, before learning to circle the *dantian*, on the following page.

*Silk Reeling exercises flow slowly and continuously. They relate to the center of the body (the* dantian*).*

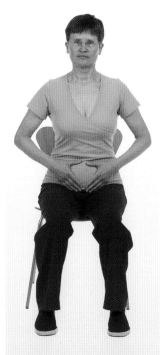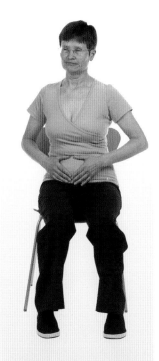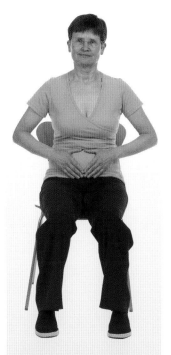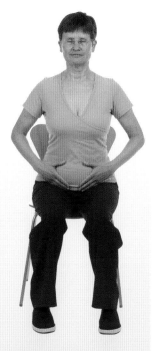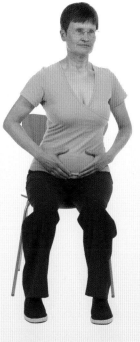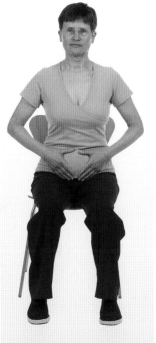

**1** Sit on a chair with your feet shoulder-width apart and the heels beneath your knees. Place your hands on the lower abdomen as shown.

**2** Keeping your head and shoulders still, rock your lower abdomen and lower back backward on the sitz bones, as if you are rolling the imaginary ball in the abdomen back over the sitz bones.

**3** With the *dantian* rocked back, twist the *dantian* slowly to the right by moving your lower abdomen. Feel as if the imaginary ball (the *dantian*) is carrying your hands around.

**4** As you slowly rock the *dantian* forward, slowly twist it to face forward.

**5** With the *dantian* rocked forward, slowly twist it to the left.

**6** As you slowly rock the *dantian* back, twist it to face forward.
Repeat steps 3–6 about 10 times, then repeat the same number of times in the opposite direction.

# Preparation—circling the *dantian*

When standing, you can move your hips freely, so in this exercise your *dantian* moves like a ball hanging from a rope that is slowly swinging around in a circle. In addition to being a *dantian* exercise, these movements also help coordinate free hip movement.

At first, make all movements slow and deliberate. Feel the hips just hanging from the *dantian* and being moved around. Once you can feel your *dantian* moving your hips in a smooth circle, experiment with increasing the speed of your movement—but don't hurry; the aim is to feel the hips moving freely.

**SIDE VIEW**

This view shows clearly how the pelvis is swung smoothly and slowly forward and back in this exercise. Follow the steps below and refer to this series to correct your position, if necessary. Keep the movement easygoing.

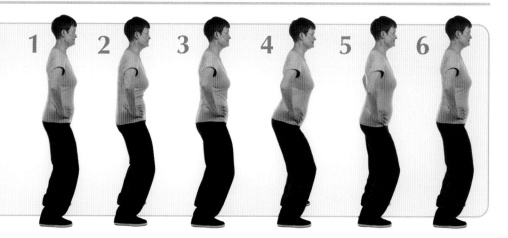

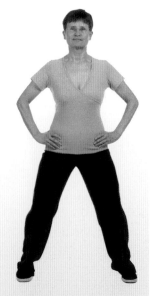

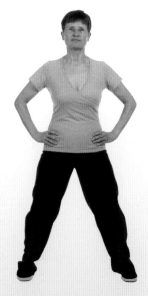

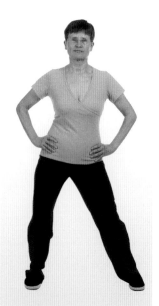

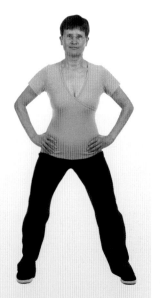

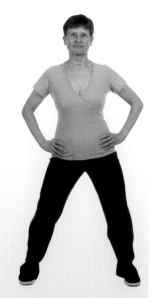

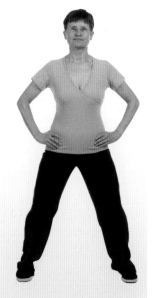

**1** Start in the Basic Posture. Place your hands on your hips. Picture your *dantian* as a ball tethered at the top.

**2** Slowly and smoothly swing the *dantian* forward so that the pelvis tilts backward.

**3** Slowly swing the *dantian* to the right (tilting the pelvis to the left).

**4** Swing the *dantian* back (tilting the pelvis forward).

**5** Swing the *dantian* to the left (tilting the pelvis to the right).

**6** Swing the *dantian* forward again. Repeat steps 3–6 about 10 times, then repeat in the opposite direction.

# Single-Hand Silk Reeling in motion

The *dantian* exercises will have prepared you for Silk Reeling. Here is one complete circle of a Single-Hand Silk Reeling movement, performed on the right side. See the flow of the movement. Try it out and repeat it a few times to get a feel for the movement. Don't worry about the precise details yet—you will learn these on the following pages.

When you start Silk Reeling, make large and expansive movements, putting emphasis on relaxation. Later, as you gain confidence with the movements and feel comfortable with them, gradually make the spirals smaller. Smaller spirals will increase your body's cohesion and allow the strength to flow more efficiently.

Remember to keep your body, especially your joints, relaxed. This will allow the spiraling movement to travel freely through the body. However, to transmit strength efficiently during the movement, you should not let your joints become lax or your body limp.

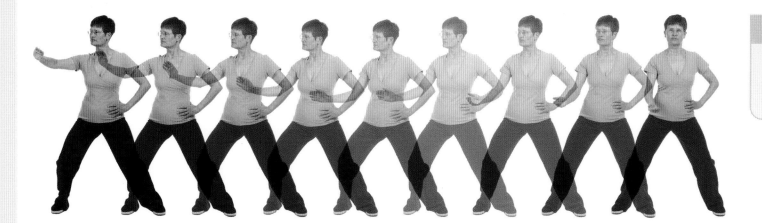

### AVOID TENSION

While learning Silk Reeling, make sure your body remains comfortable but alert, with no tension.

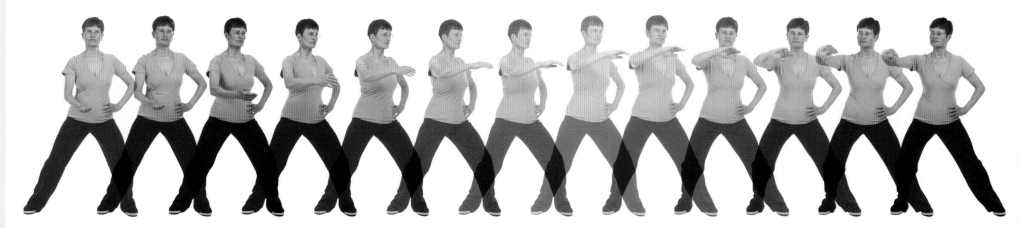

# Single-Hand Silk Reeling—moving arms and hands

To help you learn Single-Hand Silk Reeling, we have broken down the movements. First you learn how to move your arms and hands. When you can do this competently, go on to focus on how to transfer body weight and finally how to correctly turn the body. You will then be ready to combine these into a whole body movement (see page 63).

While learning the hand and arm movements, remember to keep your shoulder blades quiet and, if possible, flat across your back. If necessary, review the shoulder exercise in Chapter 2 (see page 20). Make the movements slow, continuous, and flowing.

To start with, your eyes should follow the moving hand. When you become familiar with the movement, keep your eyes level and follow only the direction of your hand with your eyes, staying aware of your hand only through peripheral vision.

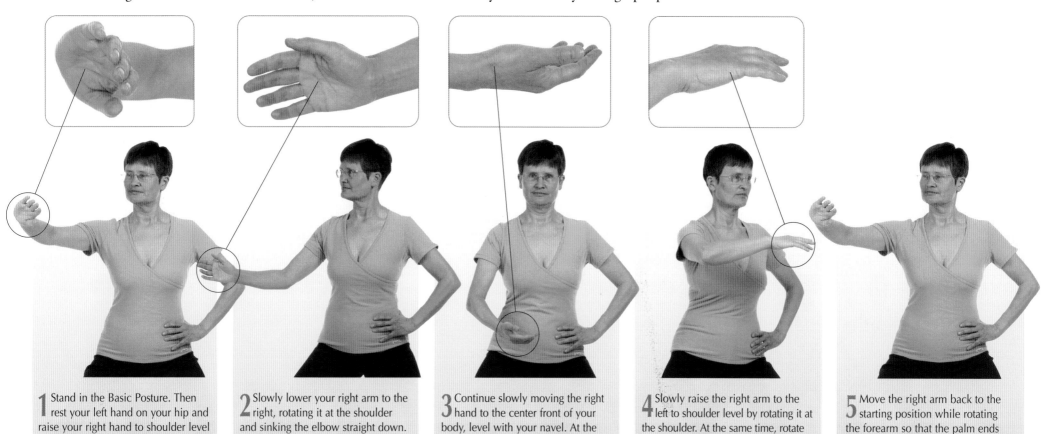

1 Stand in the Basic Posture. Then rest your left hand on your hip and raise your right hand to shoulder level in front of you, with the palm facing right and the fingers pointing forward (see page 62 for a side view).

2 Slowly lower your right arm to the right, rotating it at the shoulder and sinking the elbow straight down. At the same time, slowly turn the forearm so that the palm is facing forward as it reaches waist level.

3 Continue slowly moving the right hand to the center front of your body, level with your navel. At the same time, slowly rotate the forearm to bring the palm faceup as it reaches the center.

4 Slowly raise the right arm to the left to shoulder level by rotating it at the shoulder. At the same time, rotate the forearm so that the palm is facing down as it reaches shoulder level.

5 Move the right arm back to the starting position while rotating the forearm so that the palm ends facing right.
Repeat 10 times, then practice the same movements with the left arm.

# Single-Hand Silk Reeling—transferring your weight

During Single-Hand Silk Reeling your weight is always distributed roughly 60–40; in other words, 60 percent on the weighted leg and 40 percent on the unweighted leg.

To transfer your weight from the right leg to the left, first relax the left hip and feel as if the hip is starting to slide toward the left foot, slowly and smoothly transferring the weight onto the left leg. Do not push with the right leg. Keep the hips level, and do not move them up or down. Try to keep the knees in one place and position the hips as if you are about to sit down.

Transfer your weight from the left leg to the right in the same way.

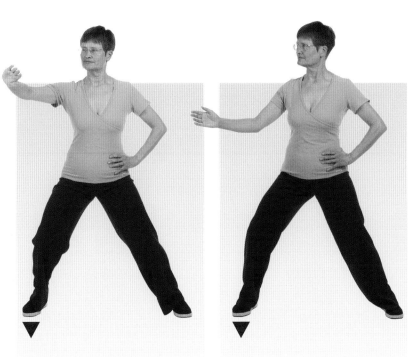 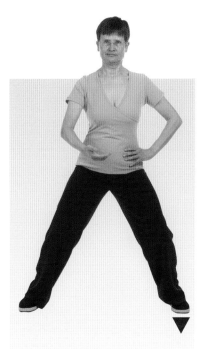 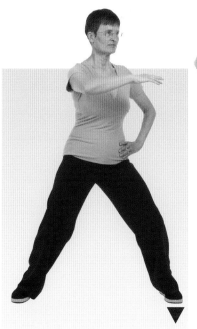 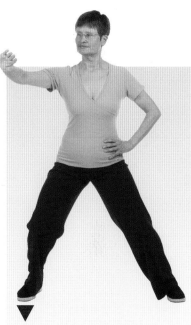

1 Start in the Horse Stance (see page 41) with 60 percent of your weight on the right foot. (Throughout these steps, concentrate on shifting your body weight while moving your arms in the way you learned on page 60.)

2 Relax the right hip and leg, and feel your weight sink through the right leg into the floor.

3 Relax the left hip, and slowly and smoothly slide the body toward the left foot as you transfer 60 percent of your weight to the left.

4 Relax the left hip and leg, and feel your weight sink through the left leg into the floor.

5 Relax the right hip, and slowly and smoothly slide the body toward the right foot as you transfer 60 percent of your weight to the right.
Repeat steps 2–5 about 10 times. Then practice the same movement on the left side.

# Single-Hand Silk Reeling—turning the body

In Silk Reeling the body turns as a result of turning the *dantian*. Turning the *dantian* not only turns the body, it also produces spirals in the body, arms, and legs and eventually creates the whole process of Silk Reeling.

The movements below are exactly the same as those shown on pages 60 and 61, but they are shown in side view to demonstrate more clearly how the body turns during the movement.

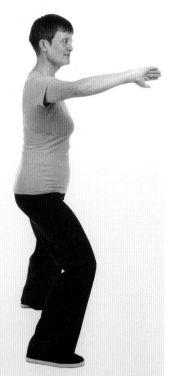

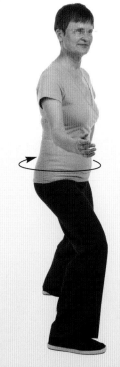

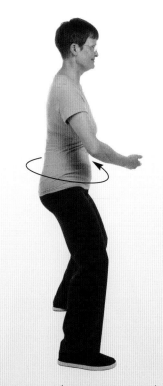

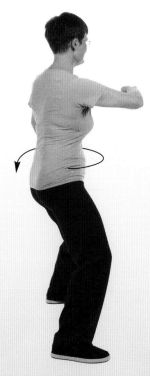

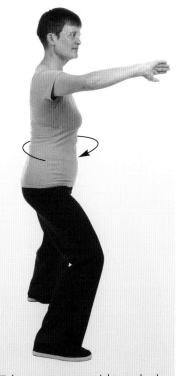

**1** Start with the body facing forward. (Throughout the following steps, concentrate on your body turning while moving your arms and shifting your weight as you learned on pages 61 and 62.)

**2** Turn the *dantian* (with the rest of the body moving with it) to the right by pushing the right groin backward. Since you keep your knees still, the right groin becomes closed and the left one becomes open. At the end of the turn, your body is facing slightly to the right.

**3** As your right arm moves toward the center, start transferring your weight by moving the right hip, and almost immediately start opening the right groin so that as you slide to the left, you slowly turn the *dantian*. At the end of the turn, your body is facing forward.

**4** Turn your *dantian* (with the rest of the body moving with it) to the left by pushing the left groin backward. Since you keep your knees still, the left groin becomes closed and the right one becomes open. At the end of the turn, your body is facing slightly to the left.

**5** As you move your right arm back to the starting position, slowly transfer your weight by moving the left hip and opening the left groin so that as you slide to the right, you slowly turn the *dantian* to the front.

Repeat steps 2–5 about 10 times. Then practice these movements on the left side.

# Single-Hand Silk Reeling—integrated movement

Combine the arm movements, weight transference, and body turning you learned on pages 60–62 to perform Single-Hand Silk Reeling. Refer to the pictures on page 59, if necessary.

Follow these steps to learn how to integrate the movements you have learned; then go to page 64 for tips on how to improve your practice.

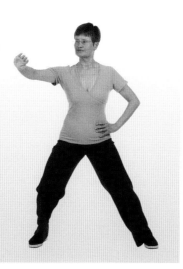

**1** Face forward in the Horse Stance with 60 percent of your weight on the right foot. Rest your left hand on the hip. Raise your right hand to shoulder level in front of you, with palm facing right and fingers pointing forward.

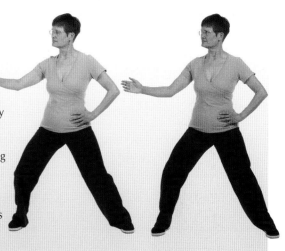

**2** Keeping your knees still, relax the right hip and leg, and feel your weight sink through the right leg into the floor as you slowly turn your body slightly to the right. At the same time, slowly lower the right arm to the right, rotating it at the shoulder, and sink the elbow straight down, turning the forearm so that the palm is facing forward as it reaches waist level.

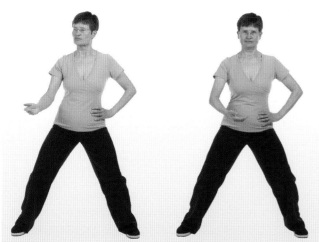

**3** Slowly turn your body to face forward as you transfer 60 percent of your weight to the left leg. At the same time, continue slowly moving the right hand to the center front of your body, level with your navel, as you slowly rotate the forearm to bring the palm face up as it reaches the center.

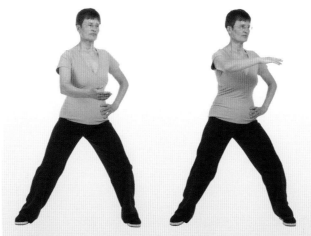

**4** Keeping knees still, relax the left hip and leg, and feel your weight sink through the left leg into the floor as you slowly turn your body slightly to the left. At the same time, slowly raise the right arm to the left to shoulder level, rotating it at the shoulder, turning the forearm so that the palm faces down as it reaches shoulder level.

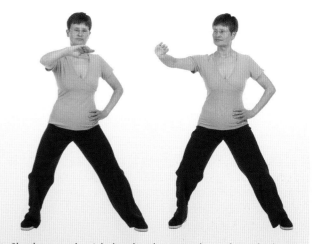

**5** Slowly move the right hand to the center front of your body. At the same time, rotate the forearm to bring the palm faceup as it reaches the center.

Repeat steps 2–5 about 10 times. Then practice Single-Hand Silk Reeling on the left side.

# Single-Hand Silk Reeling—improving movement

If you practice Single-Hand Silk Reeling correctly, after a period of practice the body, arms, and legs will move in a spiraling motion.

To achieve correct movement, you need to be patient, move softly and slowly, and pay close attention to how you are positioning and moving your body. At first, practice Silk Reeling with an emphasis on relaxation. The next step is to feel the *dantian* follow the movement of the circling hand (for example, feel as if your navel is tracking your hand).

Once you feel the *dantian* moving, you will notice that your legs are being twisted (keeping your knees facing in the same direction helps). With practice, the sensation of twisting will become clearer.

Gradually, try to feel the *dantian* pull the circling hand and the body around. Feel as if you are moving through water—your arms are floating with no effort, but at the same time, you feel a slight resistance to all your movements. The imagined resistance will make your arms lag behind the *dantian*, and this will start to create the spirals in your arms. Similarly, if you keep the body soft so that it moves in an elastic manner, the drag of the arms will start to create the spirals in your body.

Slowly start integrating the spirals into one spiraling action of the whole body, with the spirals starting from and returning to the *dantian*.

In Single-Hand Silk Reeling, the transition from position 1 through 2 to 3 (shown below) consists of a spiraling motion toward the *dantian*, and the transition from position 3 through 4 to 5 consists of a spiraling motion away from the *dantian*. As you practice the Silk Reeling exercise, follow these directions.

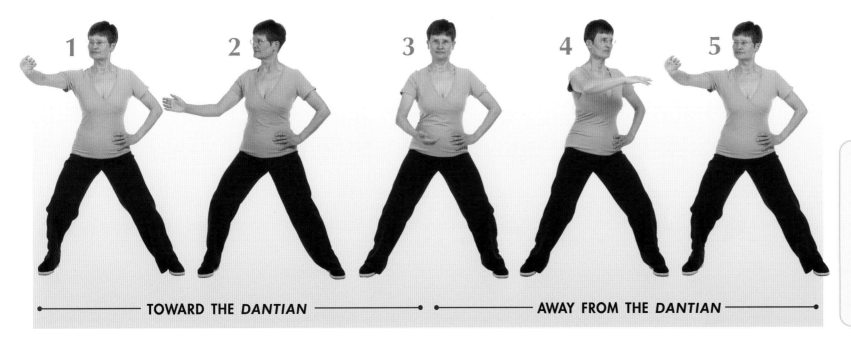

1  2  3  4  5

TOWARD THE *DANTIAN* ● ● AWAY FROM THE *DANTIAN*

### ADVANCED SILK REELING

After you have begun to practice the Tai Chi Form, you will be able to improve your Silk Reeling even further. In Chapter 9 we move Silk Reeling to a higher level of Tai Chi.

# Reverse Single-Hand Silk Reeling

Once you have mastered Single-Hand Silk Reeling, it's time to learn the reverse version. The leg and body movements are exactly the same as for the Single-Hand Silk Reeling. The arm circles in the opposite direction, but the hand positions and the twisting directions are also the same.

Step 1 and the final positions in steps 2, 3, and 4 all correspond to the same four steps for Single-Hand Silk Reeling. Then the last posture for both is returning to the starting position.

Follow the steps here, keeping in mind what you have learned about hand and arm movements, transferring weight, and body turning. Repeat the practice first with the right arm and hand as pictured, then with the left arm and hand.

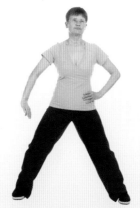

**1** Start as for Single-Hand Silk Reeling, but lower your right arm, with the palm facing to the right and the fingers pointing diagonally forward and down.

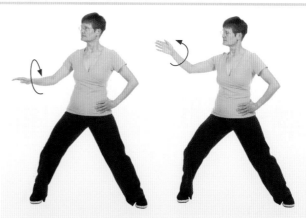

**2** Slowly raise your right arm to the right to shoulder level, rotating it at the shoulder and sinking the elbow straight down. At the same time, slowly turn the forearm so that the right palm is facing forward as it reaches shoulder level.

## HAND POSITIONS

Here are close-ups of the hand positions for the final posture in each step.

They are all in the Tai Chi Palm position (see page 43). Keep the hands comfortable and relaxed, but not limp.

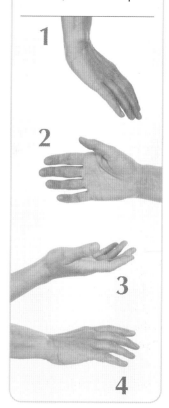

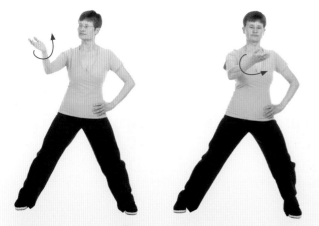

**3** Slowly move the right hand to the center front of your body. At the same time, rotate the forearm to bring the palm faceup as it reaches the center.

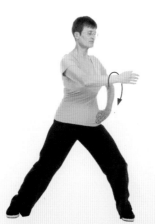

**4** Slowly move the right arm to the left as you lower it to waist level, rotating it at the shoulder. At the same time, slowly rotate the forearm to bring the right palm facedown as it reaches waist level.

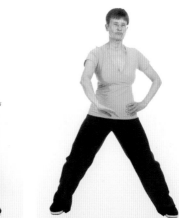

**5** Move the right arm to the right, back to the starting position, while rotating the forearm so that the palm ends facing right as in step 1.

# Double-Hand Silk Reeling

Double-Hand Silk Reeling is a combination of the Single-Hand and Reverse Single-Hand Silk Reeling. (Do not attempt this movement until you have mastered Single-Hand and Reverse Single-Hand Silk Reeling with both right and left arms.) The right arm follows the pattern for Single-Hand Silk Reeling (see page 63), while the left arm follows Reverse Single-Hand Silk Reeling (see page 65). As well as moving the arms in a clockwise direction as shown here, practice moving them counterclockwise.

Notice that as the spiral of one arm is winding toward the *dantian*, the spiral of the other is winding out from the *dantian*.

You will be using Double-Hand Silk Reeling as part of the Form in Chapter 7.

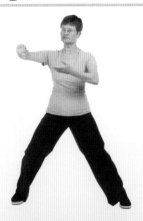
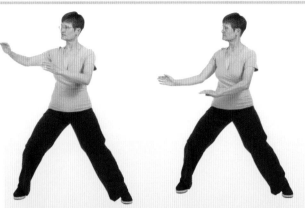
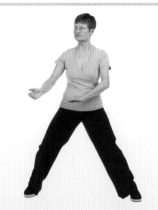

**1** Start with the right hand at shoulder level, with the palm facing right, and the left hand at the center of the body, with the palm faceup.

**2** Slowly lower the right arm to the right, turning the forearm so that the palm is facing forward as it reaches waist level, then start moving it toward the center. At the same time, lower the left arm to the center front of the body, turning the forearm to bring the palm facedown as it reaches waist level. While moving the arms, turn the body first slightly to the right then slowly toward the front.

## IMPROVE THE MOVEMENT

As you do this exercise, imagine that your arms are connected through the shoulders, and slowly shift the connection to the *dantian*. After practicing this for several weeks, you will feel the spiral of each arm joining into one movement.

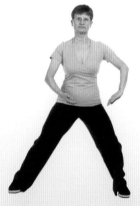
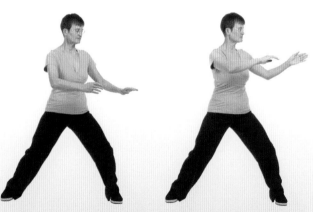
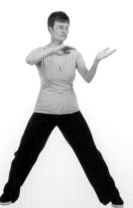
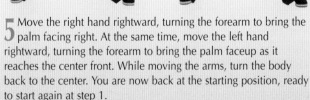

**3** Move the right arm to the center front. At the same time, move the left arm to the left, with the palm facing to the right and the fingers pointing down.

**4** Slowly raise the right arm up to the left, turning the forearm so that the palm faces down as it reaches shoulder level. At the same time, raise the left arm up to the left, turning the forearm so that the right palm is facing forward as it reaches shoulder level. While moving the arms, turn the body to the left.

**5** Move the right hand rightward, turning the forearm to bring the palm facing right. At the same time, move the left hand rightward, turning the forearm to bring the palm faceup as it reaches the center front. While moving the arms, turn the body back to the center. You are now back at the starting position, ready to start again at step 1.

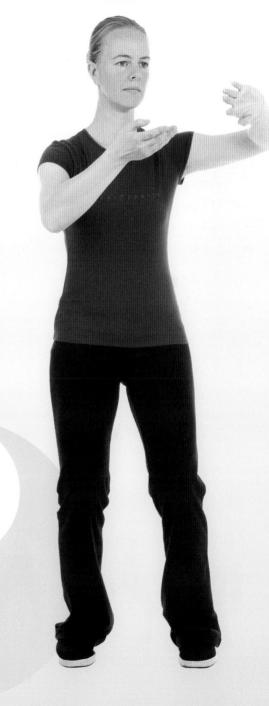

# 6 Postures for the Form

The Tai Chi Form is a flowing sequence of movements built up from linking individual exercises. In this chapter you will learn the static postures that will eventually make up the Form. They are exercises in themselves, and learning to hold these postures will relax and strengthen your body and prepare you for performing the Form.

*Controlling the breath causes strain. If too much energy is used, exhaustion follows.*

—FROM *Dao De Jing* BY LAO TZU

When people think of Tai Chi, the first image is often the flowing sequence of movements of the Form. Although the Form is the main training method, the individual components are equally important.

The postures in this chapter include all the exercises used in the Form. In the next chapter you will learn how to link these postures.

## Which Form?

There are a number of different Tai Chi schools, and each one has its own Form. However, the principles are the same no matter what the style, so all Forms are immediately recognizable as Tai Chi. The Form taught in this book is the first part of the Chen Style Laojia (Old Style) Form (see pages 141–142). The series of movements used in this Form are given in the box on this page. If you continue to practice Tai Chi, you might want to learn other Forms, but this one was chosen because it will give you a very good foundation for any future practice.

## Learning to hold postures

To learn the static postures in this chapter, follow all the instructions carefully. Teach yourself how to relax into each position and hold it with minimal effort. Only when you can do this will you be ready to start performing the movements that link the postures into one continuous Form.

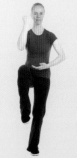

Jin Gang Pounds Mortar

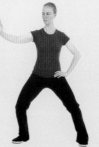

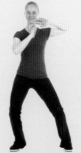

Lazy Tying Coat

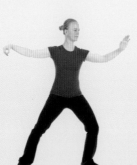

Six Sealings Four Closings

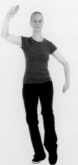

Single Whip

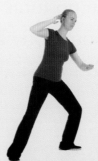

White Crane Spreads Its Wings

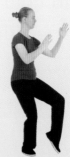

Move Sideways

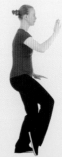

Brush Knee

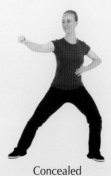

Three Steps Forward

Concealed Punch

# Central Equilibrium and awareness

Central Equilibrium is a key concept in Tai Chi theory, and it is an ongoing goal. It takes many years to achieve the perfect balance in all directions and the centered feeling that the term implies. Before starting on the postures, you need to understand its importance and learn how to move toward it.

To start on the path to Central Equilibrium, try to feel light in the upper body and "sunk down" and heavy in the lower body. This sense of balance should be present in all postures and movement.

A good way to practice Central Equilibrium is to hold each posture for a short time, concentrating on balancing and relaxing into the position (see right).

## Awareness

As you hold each of the postures in this chapter, try to become more aware of the sensations in your body. As you pay attention to your balance, you will not only become aware of the balance of your whole body but also of the individual parts of your body (see far right).

The more aware you become, the easier it will be to let go of tension in your body or mind. The more aware you become, the easier it will be to feel the right way to move. The more aware you become, the easier it will be to develop the right kind of strength. The more aware you become, the better!

## Practicing Central Equilibrium

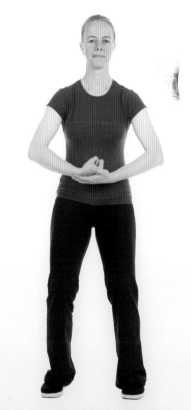

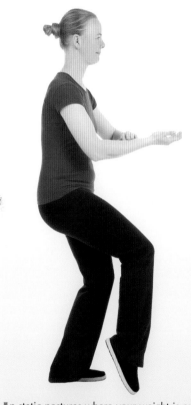

When you start to feel comfortable in a static posture, imagine that your weight is a liquid slowly draining into the ground, leaving the upper body empty.
Practice Central Equilibrium in this way as you practice each posture in this chapter.

In static postures where your weight is on one leg only, your unweighted leg should feel light and empty.

## Practicing awareness

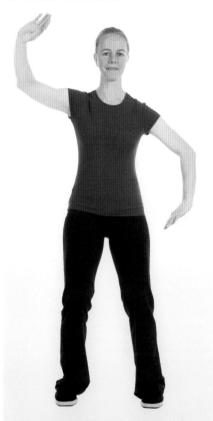

In every static posture you practice, feel your head balancing on top of your neck, the upper body balancing on top of your hips, the whole body balancing on top of your ankles. Become aware of how your body balances its weight through the spine. Feel the weight distribution on your feet but also within the body. Become aware of your skin, your muscles, and your bones.

# Beginning postures

These two postures are used as a preparation before beginning the Form. They are meant to relax your mind and body. At first glance, they may look so simple that you may think they are a waste of time, but persevere with them. If you do, you will find yourself getting more and more relaxed, and your Form practice will be more rewarding.

When you learn the Form in Chapter 7, you will learn how to move slowly and gently from posture 1 to posture 2 (see below for an explanation of posture reference numbers). For the time being, however, concentrate on how to stand correctly in each of these postures.

Hold each posture for a few minutes to experience the letting go of tension before moving on to the Jin Gang Pounds Mortar postures.

## POSTURE REFERENCE NUMBERS

The posture reference number in this chapter—P1 for posture 1, P2 for posture 2, and so on—are used for quick cross-referencing in later chapters.

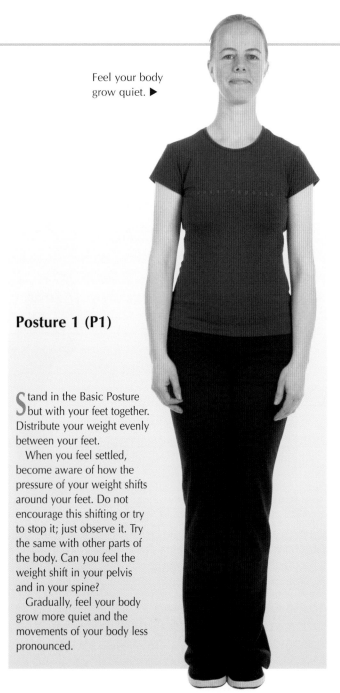

Feel your body grow quiet. ▶

### Posture 1 (P1)

Stand in the Basic Posture but with your feet together. Distribute your weight evenly between your feet.

When you feel settled, become aware of how the pressure of your weight shifts around your feet. Do not encourage this shifting or try to stop it; just observe it. Try the same with other parts of the body. Can you feel the weight shift in your pelvis and in your spine?

Gradually, feel your body grow more quiet and the movements of your body less pronounced.

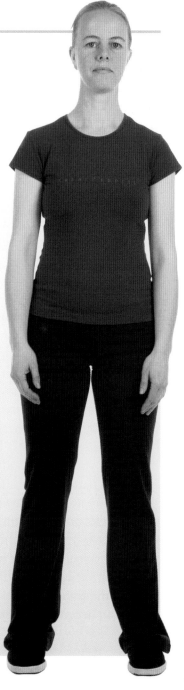

Feel steady as a mountain. ▶

### Posture 2 (P2)

Stand in the Basic Stance with your weight evenly distributed between your feet.

Be aware of your body as you did with the first posture. Notice how the weight-shifts in your feet are now much less pronounced (because of the wider base of support) and how you have to pay closer attention to feel them. Let your body grow more quiet.

Listen behind you as though you can hear faint sounds, and feel your back relax. Relax your breathing and feel your chest relax. Feel your abdomen relax. Feel calm and balanced, steady as a mountain.

# Jin Gang Pounds Mortar

Jin Gang was the name of Buddha's main bodyguard; hence, this exercise is often translated as Buddha's Attendant Warrior Pounds Mortar. The name of the movement comes from the concluding move where the fist falls into the hand as a pestle into a mortar (see P7 on page 72).

Jin Gang Pounds Mortar is repeated (with slight variations) three times in the Form. The static postures have been chosen from the first (and longest) variation, but postures 5, 6, and 7 appear in all three.

Hold each posture for about a minute, longer if you find the position easy. If a posture is strenuous, hold it for less than a minute; for example, hold postures 5 and 6 for only a short time. When your legs strengthen, especially the tendon at the top of the thigh, you will be able to hold these postures longer.

### "RIGHT" AND "LEFT" STANCES
For several postures in this chapter, you start in the Bow, Cat, and Horse Stances (see page 41). The "right" and "left" Bow or Cat Stances are named according to the leg that is forward; the "right" and "left" Horse Stances indicate the leg that is weighted.

## Posture 1 (P1)

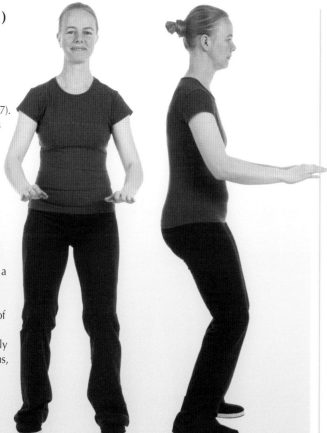

Stand in the Basic Stance (see page 17).

Move your elbows forward about 2–3 inches (5–7 cm), and raise your forearms and hands into a horizontal position with the fingers pointing forward. Feel as if your forearms and hands are resting on a big cushion.

Relax your knees and feel the weight of your body pressing your hands, especially the heels of the palms, into the cushion.

## Posture 2 (P2)

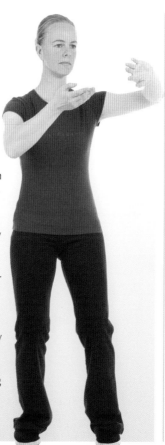

Stand in the Basic Stance. Raise your left arm so that it forms a horizontal half circle, with the palm facing out and fingertips in front of the left shoulder.

Place the right hand palm up, with the fingertips in front of the center of the chest. Keep the right elbow slightly away from the body so there is a space under the right armpit.

Shift slightly more of your weight to the right leg as you move the left hip back about an inch (2.5 cm), so that your body faces slightly left. Keep the knees pointing forward.

Feel as if you are pressing very slightly with the outward-facing palm.

## Posture 3 (P3)

Stand in the Basic Stance.

Raise your right arm so that it forms a horizontal half circle, with the palm facing out and fingertips in front of the right shoulder.

Place the left hand palm up with the fingertips in front of the center of the chest. Keep the left elbow slightly away from the body so there is a space under the right armpit.

Shift all your weight to the left leg. Keeping your left knee pointing forward, turn the body 45 degrees to the right, pivoting on the right heel and keeping the toes up. Feel as if you are pressing slightly with the outward-facing palm.

# Jin Gang Pounds Mortar—*continued*

## Posture 4 (P4)

Stand in the left Bow Stance (see page 41).

Raise your left forearm into a horizontal position with the elbow above the left knee and the hand with the palm down and fingers pointing to the right.

Rotate the right arm forward and out so that the palm is facing up and the forearm is above and parallel to the right thigh. Keep the right shoulder relaxed.

Feel as if you are resisting a weak elastic band that is linking your wrists and trying to pull them together.

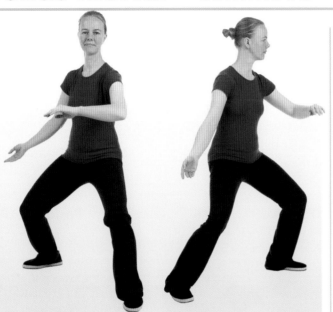

## Posture 5 (P5)

Stand in the right Cat Stance (see page 41).

Lift your right forearm forward and up to a horizontal position with palm facing up and fingers pointing forward. Lift your left forearm to a horizontal position with the hand palm down and the fingertips lightly resting on top of the right forearm as shown.

Keep both shoulders relaxed and keep a space under the armpits. The left hand should be soft and slightly cupped; the right hand should be soft and slightly stretched as if the fingers are extending forward.

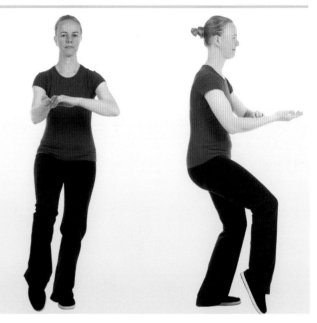

## Posture 6 (P6)

Stand in the Basic Stance. Turn the left toes slightly out and put all your weight on the left foot. Lift your right knee up, slightly higher than the hip, as you feel the right hip sink down.

Raise your right fist up above the right leg, with the right elbow hanging down. Put your left hand in front of your lower abdomen with the palm up. Keep your body upright.

Feel as if you are resisting a weak elastic band that is linking your wrists and trying to pull them together.

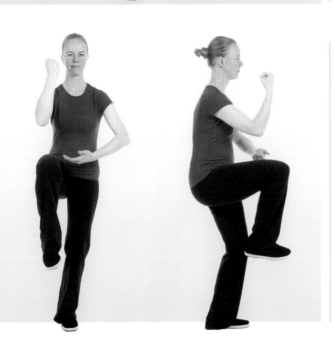

## Posture 7 (P7)

Stand in the Basic Stance. Place your hands in front of your lower abdomen with a loose right fist on top of the left palm. Your hands should not be touching the abdomen.

Keep your elbows slightly forward, widening your back.

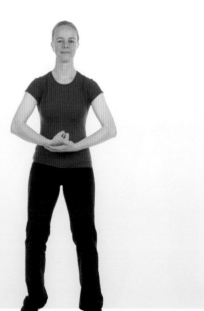
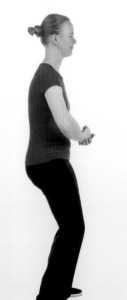

# Lazy Tying Coat

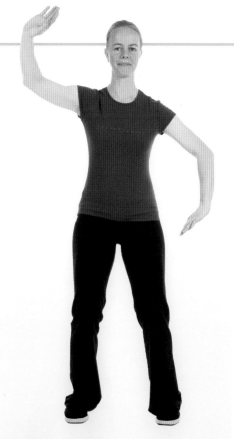

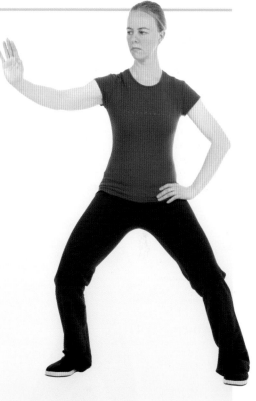

The name of this exercise comes from the way a fighter would tie the front of his long traditional Chinese coat in order to get it out of the way when he wished to fight.

These two postures should give you a very positive and open feeling. In posture 1, feel your whole body open, your shoulders and arms floating away from the body, and the intercostal spaces (between the ribs) expanding. In posture 2, try to maintain some of the open feeling while your body is settling calmly down.

Hold the postures for at least a minute until you feel relaxed.

## WORKING TO CORNERS

Some Tai Chi postures or moves are explained by describing a direction as if you were in an imaginary box and you are moving to or facing a position in the box.

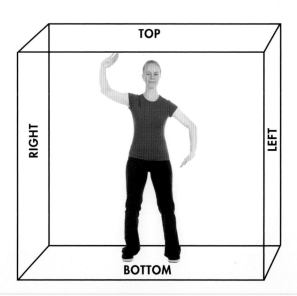

## Posture 1 (P1)

Stand in the Basic Stance. Raise your right arm so that it forms a half circle with the palm facing the front top right corner (see box left).

Rotate the left arm back and out so that the palm is facing the back lower left corner with fingers pointing in front of your feet.

Feel both arms rotating outward, but do not tighten the shoulders. Feel both hands pushing away from each other slightly. Feel that both the back and the front of the shoulders are open, as if the shoulders are being pulled very gently to the sides.

## Posture 2 (P2)

Stand in the right Horse Stance (see page 41). Raise your right arm so that the palm of the right hand faces the front right corner and the right elbow is above the right knee. Place your left hand on the left hip, fingers in front and thumb at the back. Extend the right shoulder slightly forward and feel your palm exerting a slight outward pressure.

Look over the right hand into the distance. Feel that both the back and the front of the shoulders are open, as if the shoulders are being pulled very gently to the sides.

73

# Six Sealings Four Closings and Single Whip

The names of both moves—Six Sealings Four Closings and Single Whip—are derived from their martial application. The closing move is a front push executed slightly to one side (postures 1 and 2).

The posture of the Single Whip shown here is very popular and is featured in the Forms of all styles of Tai Chi.

Hold each posture until you feel relaxed in it and any feeling of tension has been released.

## Six Sealings Four Closings

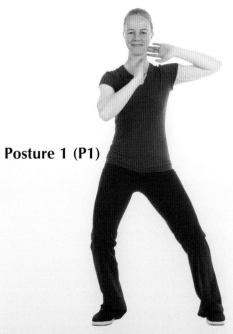

**Posture 1 (P1)**

Stand in the right Horse Stance. Raise your left arm and place the fingers of the left hand close to or touching the neck just behind the left ear. Point the left elbow to the side.

Place the fingers of the right hand close to the left thumb with the right elbow hanging down. Keep both shoulders relaxed.

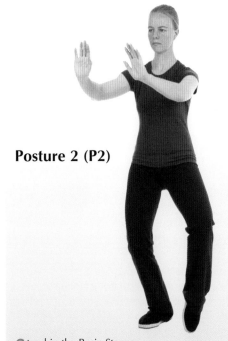

**Posture 2 (P2)**

Stand in the Basic Stance. Turn the right foot slightly to the right and lift the left heel, leaving just the tip of the big toe touching the floor.

Raise your arms and extend them as if pushing slightly to the right. Keep your palms flat and the fingers pointing up.

Look between the hands into the distance.

## Single Whip

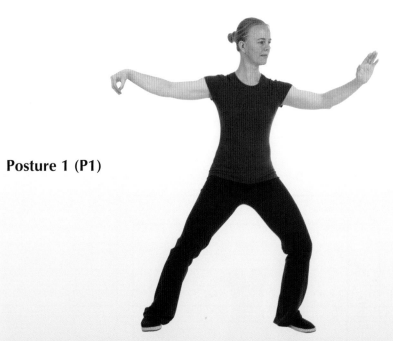

**Posture 1 (P1)**

Stand in the left Horse Stance. Form a beak with the right hand and raise it to shoulder level at the side of the body and slightly forward. Keep the arm slightly bent.

Raise the left arm to shoulder level with the left elbow above the left knee and the palm facing the front left corner (see the diagram on page 73). Extend the left shoulder slightly forward and feel your palm exerting a slight outward pressure.

Keep both shoulders relaxed and look over the left hand into the distance.

# White Crane Spreads Its Wings

**A** white crane is a traditional symbol of longevity, and this movement is often featured in breathing exercises where arm movements are used to help open the intercostal spaces between the ribs.

The name White Crane refers both to the posture of the body (resembling a crane standing on one leg and lifting a wing to cool its side) and to the movement of the back and the chest when opening and closing the arms (representing a crane's wings).

Assume the position as explained and hold it for a minute.

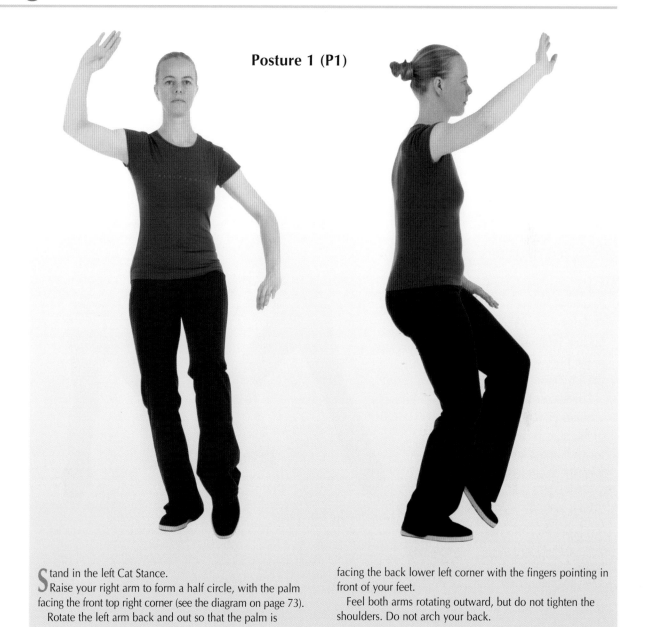

**Posture 1 (P1)**

## POSTURE TIPS

When learning this posture, keep in mind the following:

- Feel as if both hands are pushing out from the center of the palms. As a result, the hands should be slightly stretched.

- Extend your shoulders very slightly outward with your hands pushing away from each other lightly.

- At the same time, feel as if the ribs on the right side (under the right arm) are contracting lightly toward each other and exerting a very light downward pull on the right shoulder.

**S**tand in the left Cat Stance.
Raise your right arm to form a half circle, with the palm facing the front top right corner (see the diagram on page 73).
Rotate the left arm back and out so that the palm is facing the back lower left corner with the fingers pointing in front of your feet.

Feel both arms rotating outward, but do not tighten the shoulders. Do not arch your back.

75

# Move Sideways

Move Sideways is performed twice in slightly different variations within the Form (see pages 95–96 and 99–100). Below are two postures that appear in both versions.

As for all the postures in this chapter, hold each one for about a minute. Move Sideways posture 1 is unusual in Tai Chi because it is slanted; do your best to feel balance in the body while holding it. If you find it too difficult to hold for as long as a minute, hold it just long enough to become as relaxed as you can in the position. If you sense tension creeping in, move out of the position.

### Posture 1 (P1)

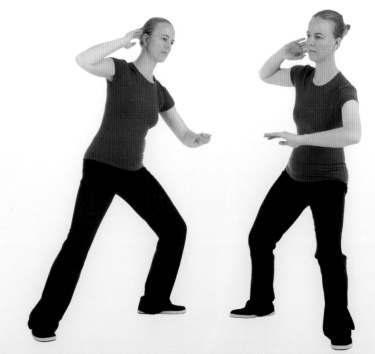

### Posture 2 (P2)

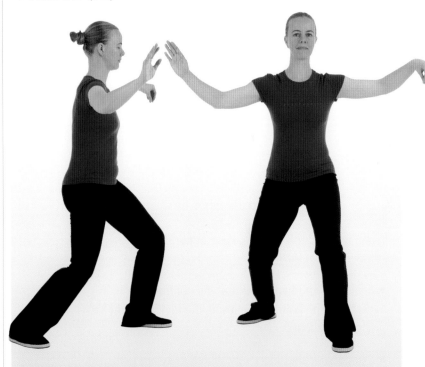

## POSTURE TIPS

The key to attaining these postures is to keep the hips loose and relaxed. The first posture requires the weight of the body to sink through the left hip into the left leg.

The second posture requires enough flexibility in the hips to face them forward and align them with the shoulders.

Stand in the left Bow Stance.
Turn to the right and lower the left hip so that you lean to the left until the right leg, the body, and the head are all in one line.

Position the left elbow above the left knee, with the forearm horizontal, palm facing down, and fingers pointing to the right of the left leg. Position the right hand above the shoulder with the palm facing your ear.

Feel as if you are balancing something on your right shoulder.

Stand in the left Bow Stance.
Open your arms to the sides with the hands at shoulder level and slightly forward. Slightly bend both arms, with the elbows pointing down, the left hand forming a beak, and the right hand open with the palm facing the front right corner (see the diagram on page 73).

The hips and the body should face directly forward; this is often very difficult due to tight hip flexors.

Make sure the lower back doesn't arch.

# Brush Knee and Three Steps Forward

The postures selected for these two exercises are excellent for training your balance. When lifting or moving a leg, it is natural to focus on the moving leg. However, learning to focus on the foot of the supporting leg will improve your balance. Train yourself to mentally sink into the supporting leg.

The Brush Knee movement is used twice in the Form (see pages 97 and 100) and is performed in exactly the same way each time. Three Steps Forward also appears twice, but in slightly different variations (see pages 98 and 101).

## POSTURE TIP

Imagine the weight of your upper leg slowly draining like a liquid into the supporting leg. One leg feels like a feather, floating in the air; the other one feels like a heavy anchor, fixing you to the floor.

## Brush Knee

### Posture 1 (P1)

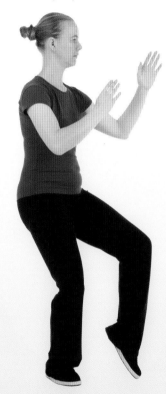

Stand in the left Cat Stance.
Raise both hands in front of your chest, with the left hand slightly higher than the right one and the palms facing each other.

Feel as if you are gently squeezing a ball of cotton wool between your hands.

## Three Steps Forward

### Posture 1 (P1)

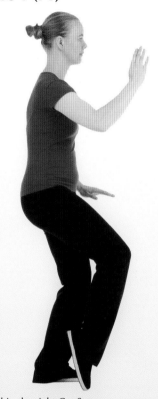

Stand in the right Cat Stance.
Lift the right knee so that the toes just clear the floor, and suspend the foot close to the left ankle.

Raise the right hand in front of you and above the shoulder, with the palm facing left and slightly toward your face and the elbow hanging down.

Raise the fingers of the left hand forward so that the left palm faces down.

Focus on your weight settling down into the left foot.

### Posture 2 (P2)

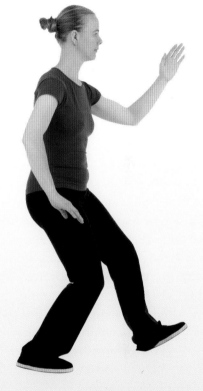

Stand in posture 1 of Brush Knee (see far left).
Lift the left leg and place the heel forward and down on the floor, keeping all the weight on the right leg.

Extend the left arm forward a little, and lower your right arm so that the right hand is by your right hip joint.

Feel your hands pushing away from each other slightly.

# Concealed Punch

When punching, most people think of using the arms. What you need to train here is the strength of the leg flowing into the punching arm.

Practice holding each of these postures first, as you did for the other postures in this chapter. Then, to better prepare yourself for learning the Concealed Punch in the Form (see page 102), practice moving between the two postures as follows: Starting in posture 1, imagine pushing a fairly big weight with your right fist, feeling the reactive force traveling into your right foot. Slowly transfer the weight to the left leg as you move into posture 2, at the same time feeling the force coming from the right leg. After holding posture 2 for a while, slowly reverse into posture 1. As you withdraw the right arm, feel that the movement compresses your right leg. Feel the compression in the right leg as you hold posture 1. After a while repeat the cycle again.

## MOVEMENT TIP

While the right leg provides the strength, the left elbow provides the speed. The faster you pull the left elbow back, the faster the right fist will shoot forward.

**Posture 1 (P1)**

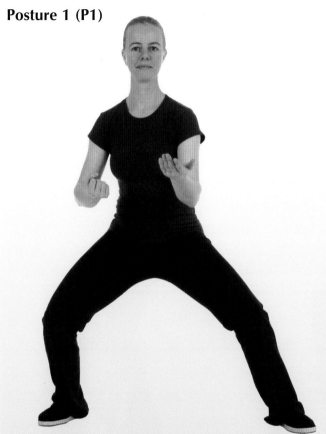

Stand in the left Bow Stance.
Transfer your weight to the right leg and turn your body to the right.

Raise the forearms to a horizontal position by the sides of the body. Position the left arm slightly more forward than the right one, with both arms pointing in the same direction as the right foot, the left hand open with the palm facing up, and the right hand palm up and closed into a soft fist.

Feel as if you are trying to turn the body to the left but there is a resistance behind the left elbow and in front of the right fist, preventing you from moving.

**Posture 2 (P2)**

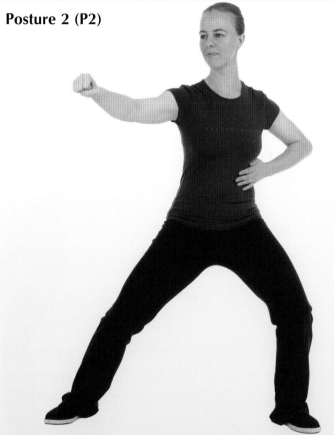

Stand in the left Bow Stance.
Face the hips in the direction of the left foot. Raise the right arm to shoulder level with the hand in a fist and the palm facing down.

Touch the lower left ribs with the palm of the left hand.

Keep the right hand soft, the right elbow slightly bent, and the right shoulder sunk down.

Look above the right hand into the distance.

Feel as if you are stretching the right fist and the left elbow away from each other.

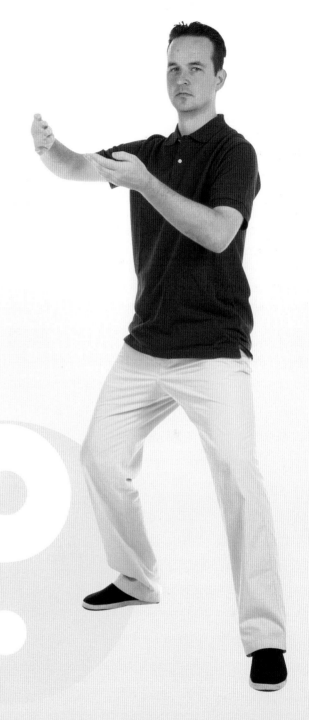

# 7 Learning the Form

Now that you have practiced the static postures, you are ready to link them into the slow, flowing movement of the Form.

*In stillness, stand like a mountain peak; in movement, flow like a mighty river.*

—FROM THE TAI CHI *Classics*

This chapter teaches you the simple movements of the Form. Don't worry too much about accuracy at this stage, and don't rush it. With practice you will absorb the movements of the Form from start to finish.

While learning the Form, keep in mind the posture and movement lessons you learned in Chapter 2 (see pages 11–22).

Through correct and natural balance you will be able to move slowly and smoothly without engaging your phasic muscles to provide support for your body. This is not difficult to do when moving just one part of the body, but it takes more concentration when the whole body is moving. However, with regular practice it will become automatic and feel natural.

## Individual exercises of the Form

In Chapter 6 you were introduced to each exercise in the Form. Learn and become familiar with each exercise and its series of movements before moving on to the next. Follow the steps in the box on the right as a guide to practice.

After you have learned all the exercises one at a time in the order given in this chapter, you will be able to link them together in the slow, continuous motion of the Form, which takes three to five minutes from start to finish.

### HOW TO LEARN EACH EXERCISE

**1.** Try the individual moves of the exercise, making sure you can perform them comfortably. Make no effort to memorize the movements at this stage.

**2.** Start in the first position and hold it for a while. Focus on your balance and the sensation as your joints relax and your body settles down. Keeping relaxed and balanced, slowly and softly move into the next position. Repeat the movement several times to memorize it and to improve it. Be aware of the sensations in different parts of your body.

**3.** Repeat step 2 with each movement in the exercise.

**4.** Once you can confidently perform the individual movements, link them together to perform the whole exercise. Repeat the exercise several times, moving more softly and smoothly each time and becoming more aware of the sensations in your body.

### Six Sealings Four Closings
The fourth exercise in the Form.

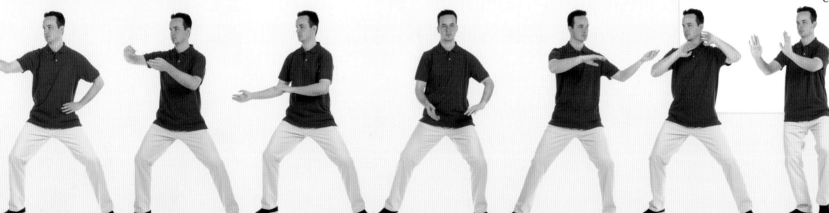

# How to overcome difficulties

If you find that a movement is too difficult while you are learning the Form, pinpoint the problem and follow the tips here to overcome it. You are in charge! The overriding principle at this stage is to be comfortable.

Always warm up before practice and concentrate on the areas that are stiff. With time, if you practice regularly, your body will become more flexible and the movement should become easier.

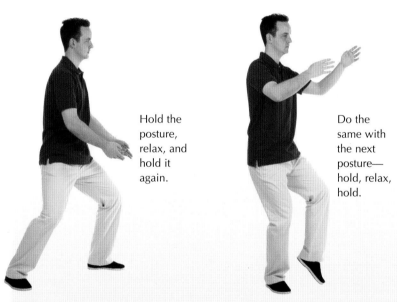

Hold the posture, relax, and hold it again.

Do the same with the next posture— hold, relax, hold.

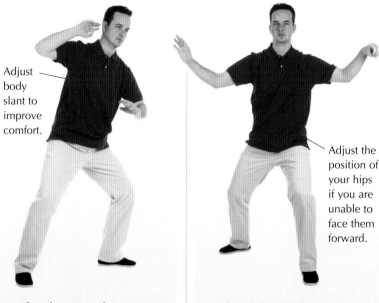

Adjust body slant to improve comfort.

Adjust the position of your hips if you are unable to face them forward.

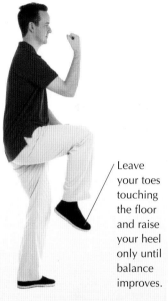

Leave your toes touching the floor and raise your heel only until balance improves.

## Poor coordination

If the source of the difficulty is poor coordination, slow down your pace of learning. Don't think of the move as complicated; think of it as a transition through a series of simple postures. Start with the posture that just precedes the problem move and hold it for a while, feeling your body relax. Adjust your posture a little and hold it again. Try this with the two postures above (from Brush Knee 1, page 97). To master an entire exercise, go through several static postures in this way, then link them in a continuous movement.

## Lack of strength

If you lack the strength for a particular position, adjust the position so that you are comfortable. For example, in Move Sideways 1 (step 5, page 96), if you feel that your legs, hips, or back are not strong enough to hold this slanted posture (shown above in side view), adjust the slant so you are more comfortable. With repetition your muscles will gradually strengthen.

## Lack of flexibility

You might lack the flexibility for a position even after warming up. For example, if your hip flexors are tight, you might be unable to face your hips forward in the Move Sideways 1 posture shown above (step 8, page 96). To overcome inflexibility, adjust the height of the hips, angle of the body, or limb position until you are comfortable. Over time, with regular practice, your body will become more flexible.

## Lack of balance

If you find it difficult to balance, adjust the posture to eliminate the problem. For example, if you keep losing your balance when you lift a leg up, as in Jin Gang Pounds Mortar, shown above (side view of step 9, page 86), lift only your heel, leaving your toes touching the floor. When this way becomes comfortable, gradually leave less weight on the toes until you are practically standing on one leg.

# Movement tips

The box below lists some key points for you to remember throughout your practice. Review these tips regularly as you are learning the Form. Gradually, they will become so automatic you will forget having had to learn them.

Now that you are ready to learn movements rather than static postures, there are two basic arm movements referred to in the Form that you will need to learn. They are called "circling" and "rotating" and they are shown on this page. Familiarize yourself with the movements before starting to learn the Form.

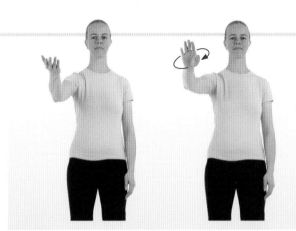

## Rotating arm in or out
To rotate out, extend an arm forward with your palm facing up, then turn the palm to face down. To rotate in, reverse the move. Make sure you rotate the whole arm, not just the forearm.

## POINTS TO WATCH

When first learning the moves of the Form, keep in mind the following points:

- Let your head float up and your weight sink down.

- Always point your knees in the same direction as your feet.

- Always keep the feeling of a round space under both armpits so that your elbows do not touch the body.

- Before you step, look in the direction of the step. Let your eyes follow the moving hand. If both hands move, follow the one that is higher.

- When you take a step away from your body, put your heel down first.

- When you take a step toward your body, put the toes down first.

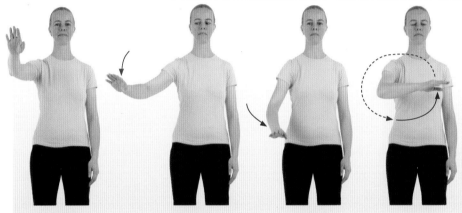

## Circling arm
To circle an arm, extend it forward and, with your hand, draw a circle in the air. Turn your waist slightly to the right as you lower your right arm by rotating it at the shoulder. Allow your elbow to sink straight downward.

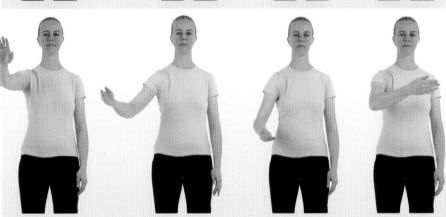

## Rotating and circling arm
Combine circling and rotation. Most arm movements in Tai Chi are a combination of circling and rotating.

# Starting the Form

Start the Form by standing with your feet together, and then move gently and calmly into the Basic Posture (see page 17).

The step can be made in either direction, to the right or left, whichever is more comfortable. As you improve your Form, you should hold the first posture for a shorter period and the second one for a longer period. Eventually, hold the first posture just to settle down, and then slowly step sideways and hold the second posture for 3–5 minutes (or longer, if you have the time).

After practicing this first move, go on to learning the exercises on the following pages.

## POSTURE REFERENCE NUMBERS

The posture reference numbers in this chapter—**P1** for posture 1, **P2** for posture 2, and so on—are for quick cross-referencing to the static postures practiced in Chapter 6.

P1

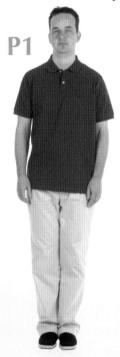
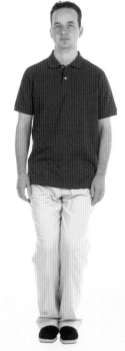
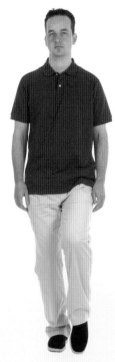
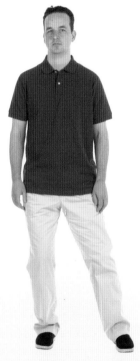

P2

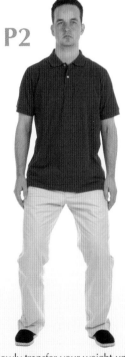

1 Stand in the Basic Posture, but with the feet together. Stand like this until you feel calm and settled (**P1**; page 70—see box on this page about reference numbers).

2 Sink your body down by letting go in your hips, knees, and ankles. Go down as far as is comfortable.

3 Keeping your hips level, lift your left heel as you shift your weight to the right leg.

4 Move your left foot to the left until your feet are shoulder-width apart. Touch the floor first with the toes of the left foot, then place the heel down, still keeping your weight on your right leg. Your left knee should remain slightly bent.

5 Slowly transfer your weight until it is equally distributed between the feet. Do this by slightly straightening the right leg, without increasing the bend in the left one, so that both knees are flexed the same amount. Calm body and mind and settle your awareness in the *dantian* (**P2**).

# 1: Jin Gang Pounds Mortar 1

## AT A GLANCE:

- Lift and lower arms.

- Circle the arms in a figure eight, pushing the left hand to the left and then the right hand to the right.

- Step forward with the left leg, then with the right, into a Cat Stance as you pierce the right fingers forward.

- Slam the right fist into the left palm as you stomp the right foot down.

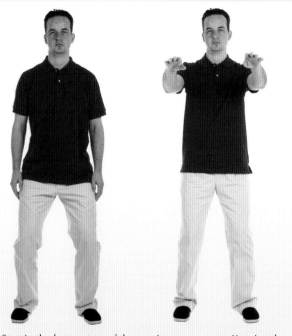
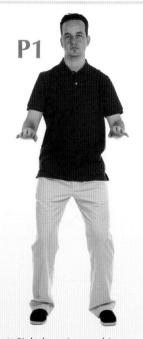
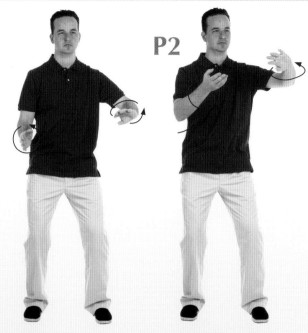

**1** Start in the last posture of the previous movement. Keeping the hands relaxed and hanging down, slowly float your arms up to shoulder level. Then slowly float your hands upward, extending the fingers forward.

**2** Sink down in your hips, letting this movement pull your arms slowly down to waist level as if they are resting on a cushion (**P1**; page 71). Let the floating up and sinking down of the arms determine the slow rhythm of the following moves.

**3** Sinking a bit more onto the right leg, turn slightly to the left. At the same time, rotate your left arm out and up until the palm faces left and the elbow is shoulder level, while the right arm follows, rotating in until the palm faces up and the fingers point toward the left fingers (**P2**).

*(continued on next page)*

## ENDING AND STARTING EXERCISES

Each exercise in the Form is started in the last posture of the previous exercise. When you become familiar with practicing the Form, you will be able to flow from one exercise into the next without stopping.

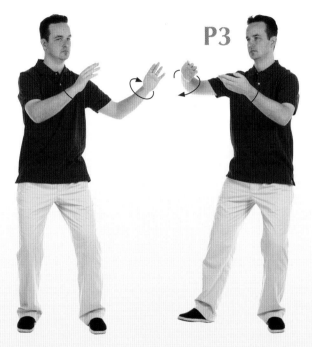

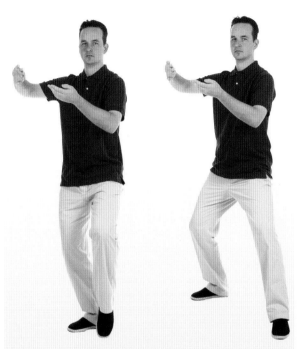

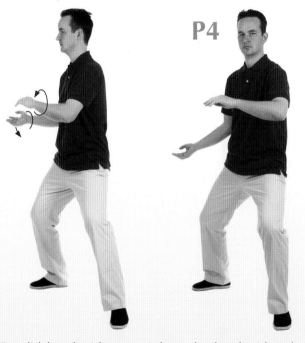

**4** Turn slightly left as you start sinking the left arm, with the elbow leading and the arm rotating in; at the same time, raise and rotate the right arm out, slightly widening the gap between the hands.

When the left forearm is again horizontal, the left hand faces forward, the right elbow is at shoulder level, and the right hand faces down, turn the whole body (except for the left leg) to the right. At the same time, continue to rotate both arms, moving the left hand gradually closer to the right hand, and transfer all your weight to the left leg.

With the right heel touching the ground, gradually lift the rest of the foot and rotate it 45 degrees to the right (**P3**). Make all movements continuous and circular.

**5** Transfer your weight to the right leg. Look forward, turning the head 45 degrees to the left as you bring the left foot close to the right one, placing just the tip of the big toe on the floor. Step with your left leg diagonally forward into a left Bow Stance, touching the floor only with your heel. Do not transfer any weight to the left leg.

**6** Turn slightly to the right as you circle your hands to the right and down, the left one rotating out and the right one in (as you learned to do for the first arm movement of Double-Hand Silk Reeling on page 66). At the same time, lower the left foot to the floor, toes pointing forward.

When both forearms are horizontal, the right palm faces toward the right, and the left palm faces down, turn the body left and transfer 60 percent of your weight to the left leg. At the same time, keep the right hand in the same place and let the movement slightly pull the right elbow so that the right palm turns upward. The left elbow ends above the left knee, which is slightly behind the left toes (**P4**).

*(continued on next page)*

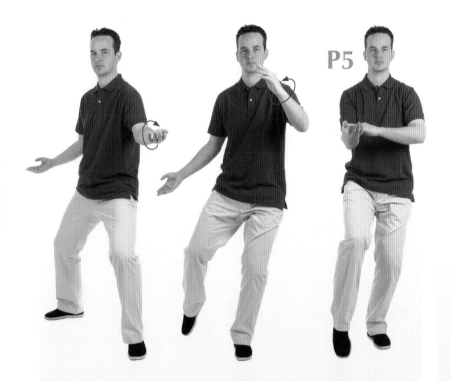

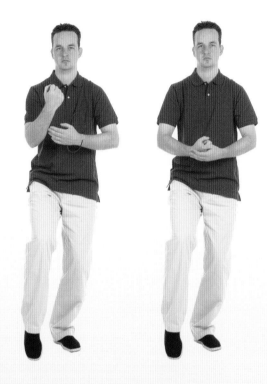

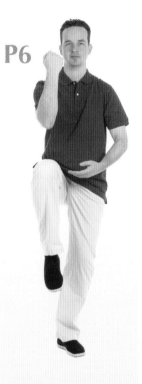

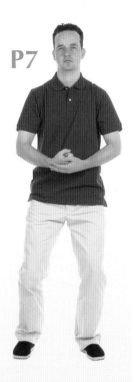

**7** Keeping the left elbow fixed, extend the left hand forward as you rotate the palm up. Continue moving the left arm up and over to the right and down while turning the arm out. As you start lowering your left arm, step forward with your right leg into the right Cat Stance and move your right arm forward, with the elbow passing close to the body until the right inside forearm touches the fingers of your descending left hand. The right palm is up and the fingers point forward; the left arm is in a horizontal position again (**P5**). When moving forward, the right arm and leg move as one.

**8** Rotate the left palm up as you make a loose fist with your right hand and place it in the left palm. Throughout this move, keep the fingers of the left hand in touch with the right forearm and pivot the right forearm around this point. As you raise the right hand up, the elbow goes down; as you move the right hand back toward the left hand, the right elbow circles forward.

**9** Lift the right knee and the right fist as one. The right forearm is vertical; the right foot hangs down (**P6**).

**10** Lift the right foot to a horizontal position, then stomp the right foot down as you slam the right fist into the left palm. The right foot should strike the floor flat as the back of the right fist slams into the left palm (**P7**).

# 2: Lazy Tying Coat

**AT A GLANCE:**

- Start by moving the right arm upward and the left arm downward. Circle your arms clockwise until the wrists cross, with the left wrist on top.

- Step to the right.

- Make a big wave, left to right, with your right hand.

*When you move correctly, the body feels as if it is floating through space. It may take some time to achieve this feeling, but that should not discourage you—that is the reason you practice!*

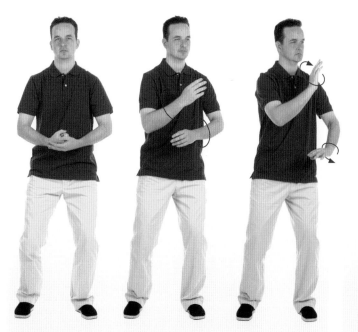

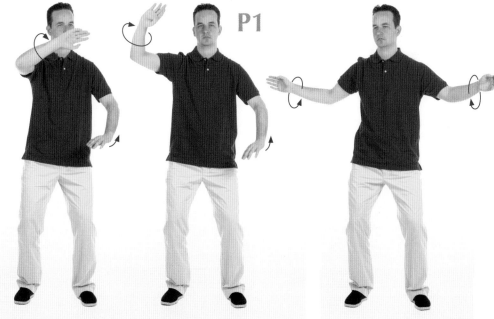

**1** Starting in the last posture of the previous movement, slowly raise the fingers of the right hand up in front of the left shoulder, using the movement to turn slightly to the left, and transfer about 60 percent of your weight to the left leg. At the same time, lower the left arm a little and rotate both arms slightly out, ending with the right palm facing the left shoulder and the left palm facing the left foot.

**2** Transfer about 75 percent of your weight to the right leg as you turn to face forward. At the same time, continue rotating the arms out and circling them—the left arm slightly more to the left and the right arm across to the right (**P1**; page 73).

**3** Transfer about 80 percent of your weight to the right leg as you turn slightly to the right, continuing to circle the arms until they are horizontal while rotating them in, with both palms facing forward.

*(continued on next page)*

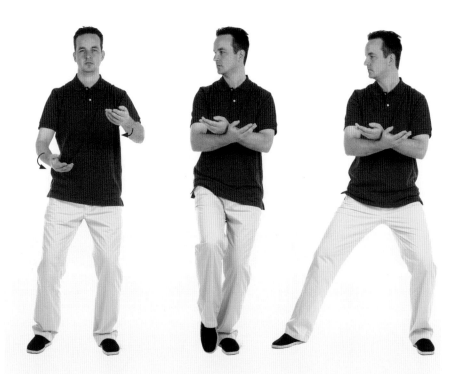

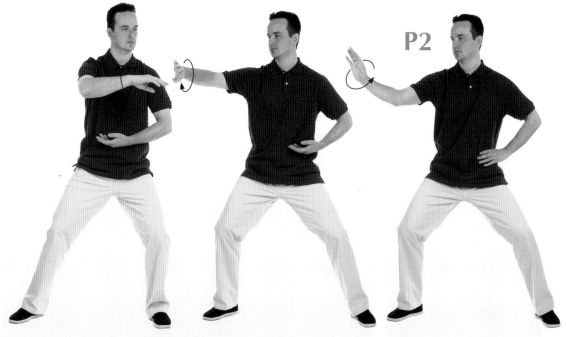

P2

4 Transfer all your weight to the left leg as you turn to face forward. Continue to circle the arms, making the circle smaller until you cross the wrists while rotating the arms in. As the wrists touch (the left wrist on top), bring your right foot next to the left foot, touching the floor only with the big toe. Look right and step to the right into a left Horse Stance, but with your right foot pointing slightly to the right (the heel touches down first).

5 Bring the fingers of the right hand up and forward in front of your left shoulder, using the movement to turn slightly to the left. Turn slightly to the right as you start rotating the right arm out. Then immediately start transferring 60 percent of your weight to the right leg as you continue turning the body to the right. At the same time, circle the right hand across to the right, still rotating the right arm out. The move ends when the right elbow is above the right knee and the right hand is in front of the right toes with the palm facing right and fingers pointing forward.

Throughout this move, keep the left hand fixed; by turning your body slightly to the right, the fixed left hand ends up in front of the left hip. Your eyes should follow the right hand.

6 Turn your body forward as you relax the hips (as if you are sitting down), and roll the shoulders back and down to relax the arms and sink the elbows. Feel the body sinking to the *dantian* (**P2**).

# 3: Six Sealings Four Closings

**AT A GLANCE:**

- Raise the left hand up to the right one.

- Circle both arms clockwise as you step to the right.

- Step the left foot in and push with both hands.

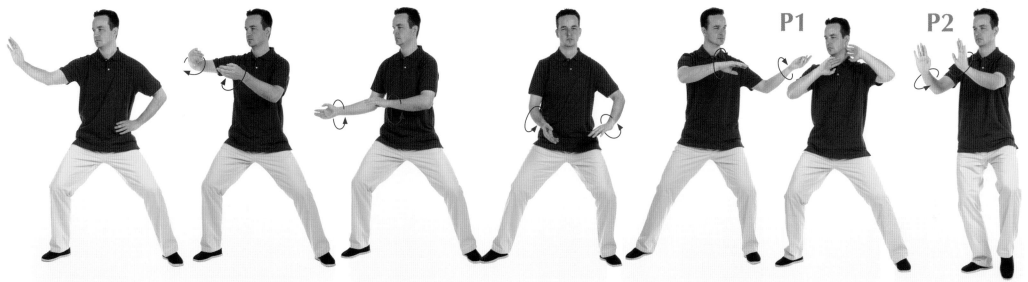

P1    P2

1 Start in the last posture of the previous movement. With the palm facing up, slowly raise the left hand toward the right hand, using the movement to turn slightly to the right. Use the turning of the body to rotate the right arm out until the elbow is at shoulder level and points sideways to the right.

2 Circle both arms clockwise as in Double-Hand Silk Reeling (see page 66) until your hands are in front of your hips.

3 Continue circling your arms, and as your hands come up on the left, raise the left hand behind your ear and the right hand just in front of the left hand. As your hands move left, transfer about 60 percent of your weight to the left leg; as your hands move right toward your neck, transfer your weight back to the right leg (**P1**; page 74).

4 Bring the left foot close to the right foot, placing only the tip of the big toe on the floor; at the same time, push your hands across your body, moving them forward and slightly to the right (**P2**).

# 4: Single Whip

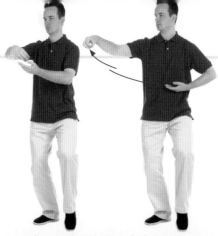
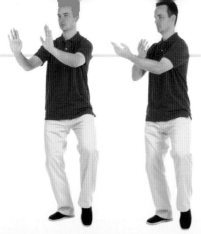
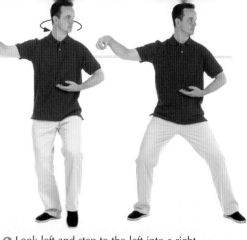

**AT A GLANCE:**

- Make a beak with the right hand.

- Step to the left.

- Make a big wave, right to left, with the left hand.

**1** Start in the last posture of the previous movement. Turn slightly to the right as you slowly rotate both hands in. Keep the right hand fixed in space, but use the movement of the body to move the left hand so that it ends up in front of the right one, with both palms facing you.

**2** Make a beak with the right hand as you rotate the right elbow out, and turn the hand so that the wrist points out and the fingers point toward your center. Turn to the left and use this movement to push the right hand to the right, shoulder level and slightly forward. At the same time, move the left hand in front of the left lower ribs.

**3** Look left and step to the left into a right Horse Stance, but with your left foot pointing slightly to the left (the heel touches down first).

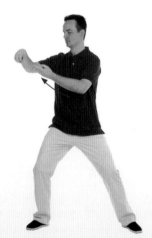
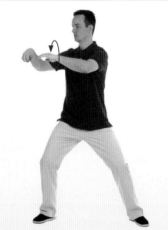
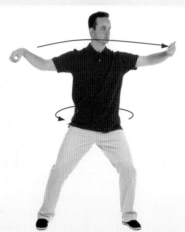
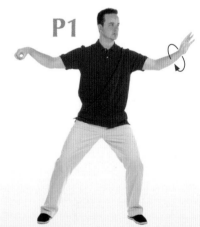

P1

**4** Raise the fingers of the left hand up and forward in front of your right shoulder, with the palm toward your face. Use this motion to turn your body slightly right as you start rotating the left arm out, then immediately start transferring 60 percent of your weight to the left leg as you turn to the left, and circle the left hand across to the left, still rotating the left arm out. The move ends when the left elbow is above the left knee and the left hand

is in front of the left toes with the palm facing left and fingers pointing forward. The body ends facing slightly left. During the shifting of your weight, when you feel most of it lifted from the right leg, turn the right foot, pivoting on the heel, until it points forward. Throughout the move, do not move the right hand. Your eyes should follow the left hand.

**5** Turn forward as you relax the hips (as if you are sitting down), and roll the shoulders back and down to relax the arms and sink the elbows. Feel the body sinking to the *dantian* (**P1**; page 74).

# 5: Jin Gang Pounds Mortar 2

## AT A GLANCE:

- Move the left hand across to the right one.

- Circle your arms clockwise in one full circle.

- Step forward with the right leg into a Cat Stance as you pierce the right fingers forward.

- Slam the right fist into the left palm as you stomp the right foot down.

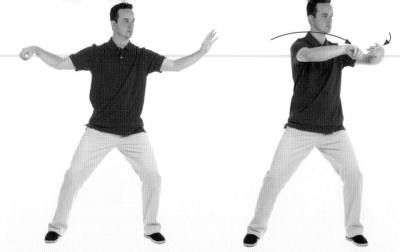

**1** Start in the last posture of the previous movement. Bring the back of the right wrist close to the left hand as you rotate both elbows out, using this movement to turn slightly to the left. Feel your back open and stretch out. The fingers of both hands point to the right.

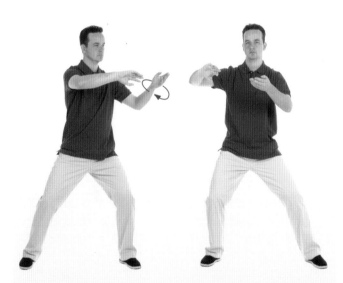

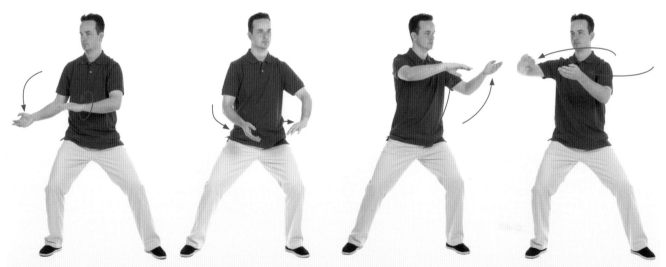

**2** Transfer 60 percent of your weight to the right leg as you turn slightly to the right, using this movement to rotate the left arm until the palm faces the right hand, which opens. Your body faces forward and your right palm faces right.

**3** Perform one full circle of a Double-Hand Silk Reeling (see page 66).

(continued on next page)

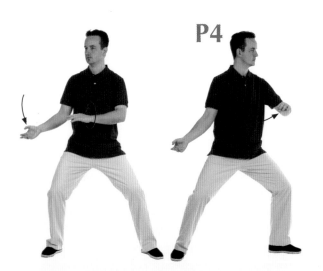
**P4**

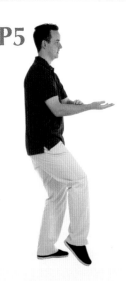
**P5**

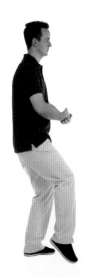

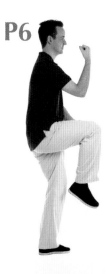
**P6**

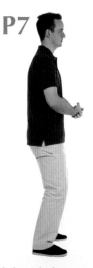
**P7**

**4** Continue circling with both hands, as in Double-Hand Silk Reeling, while you lower your right hand. Turn the body to the left 45 degrees as you transfer 60 percent of your weight to the left leg and turn the toes of the left foot to point left. At the same time as you turn the body, carry the left arm with it to the left until the elbow is above the left knee, which is slightly behind the left toes.

Keep the right hand in the same place and let the movement of the body's turning slightly pull the right elbow so that the right palm turns upward (**P4**; page 72). (See step 6 on page 85 for a view of this movement from a different angle.)

**5** Keeping the left elbow fixed, extend the left hand forward as you rotate the palm up. Continue moving the left arm up and over to the right and down while turning the arm out. As you start lowering your left arm, step forward with your right leg into the right Cat Stance and move your right arm forward, with the elbow passing close to the body, until the right inside forearm touches the fingers of your descending left hand.

The right palm is up and the fingers point forward; the left arm is in the same position from which you just started (**P5**). When moving forward, the right arm and leg move as one. (See step 7 on page 86 for a view of this movement from a different angle.)

**6** Rotate the left palm up as you make a loose fist with your right hand and place it in the left palm. Throughout this move, keep the fingers of the left hand in touch with the right forearm and pivot the right forearm around this point. As you raise the right hand up, the elbow goes down; as you move the right hand back toward the left hand, the right elbow circles forward.

**7** Lift the right knee and the right fist as one. The right forearm is vertical; the right foot hangs down (**P6**).

**8** Lift the right foot to a horizontal position, then stomp the right foot down as you slam the right fist into the left palm. The right foot should strike the floor flat as the back of the right fist slams into the left palm (**P7**).

# 6: White Crane Spreads Its Wings

## AT A GLANCE:

- Start by moving the right arm upward and the left arm downward and circle your arms clockwise until the wrists cross, with the left wrist on top.

- Step back and open your arms with an expansive movement.

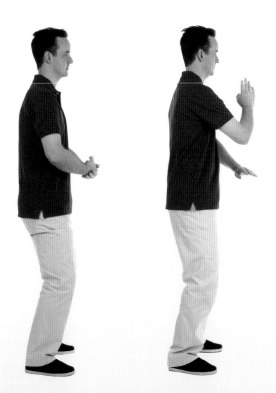
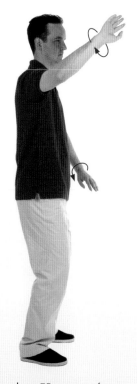
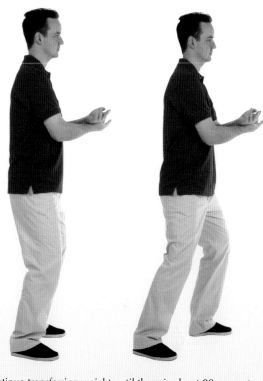

**1** Start in the last posture of the previous movement. Slowly raise the fingers of the right hand up in front of the left shoulder, using this movement to turn slightly to the left and transfer about 60 percent of your weight to the left leg. At the same time, lower the left arm a little and rotate both arms slightly out, ending with the right palm facing the left shoulder and the left palm facing the left foot. (See step 1 on page 87 for front view of this movement.)

**2** Transfer about 75 percent of your weight to the right leg as you turn back to face forward. At the same time, continue rotating the arms out and circling them—left arm slightly more to the left and the right arm across to the right. (See step 2 on page 87 for front view of this movement.)

**3** Continue transferring weight until there is about 80 percent on the right leg as you turn slightly to the right. At the same time, continue to circle the arms (while rotating them in) until they are horizontal, with both palms facing forward. As you turn to face forward, transfer all your weight to the left leg and continue to circle and rotate the arms, making the circle smaller until the wrists cross.

As the wrists touch (left wrist on top), bring your right foot next to the left foot and, without pausing, step diagonally back, keeping your weight on the front (left) leg.

*(continued on next page)*

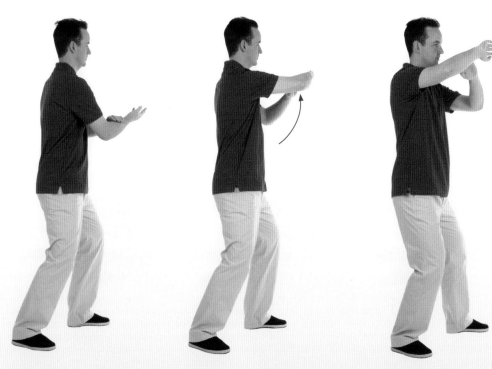

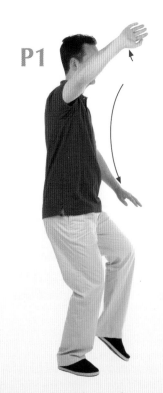

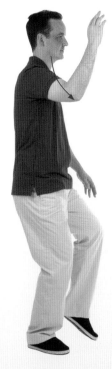

P1

4 Turn slightly left as you push the right hand toward the left front (the motion of the right arm rolls the left wrist along the right forearm), and almost immediately start rotating the right arm out (rolling it along the left hand) and transferring all your weight to the right leg as you keep turning the body to the right. End with both hands facing forward, the left fingers touching the back of the right forearm, and the body facing slightly to the left.

5 Turn to face forward, using this move to open the arms—the right arm up, with the palm facing the top front-right corner; the left arm down, with the palm facing the bottom back-left corner. Extend from the *dantian* to the fingertips of both hands (**P1**; page 75).

6 Relax the hips (as if you are sitting down), and roll the shoulders back and down to relax the arms and sink the elbows. Feel the body sinking to the *dantian*.

## AT A GLANCE:

- Push the right hand forward.

- Push the left hand forward and take a step forward with the left leg.

- Turn right and tilt to the left by sinking into the left hip.

- Turn left as you sweep your left hand in front of the left knee. Turn the left hand into a beak and raise it to shoulder level. At the same time, move your right hand past your neck and sweep it horizontally left to right.

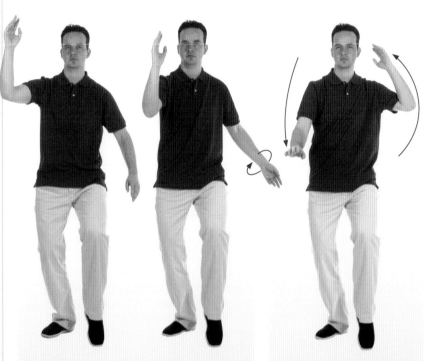

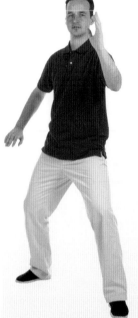

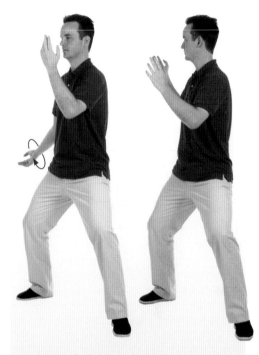

1 Start in the last posture of the previous movement. Slowly push the right hand forward with the palm facing left as you rotate the left shoulder out until your left hand faces nearly to the left.

2 Raise your left hand up and forward behind your neck in a circular motion as you move the right hand forward and down with the palm facing down.

3 Push the left hand forward with the palm facing right as you raise the right hand back to your right hip with the palm facing down. Push the left hand more forward and the right hand more back as you step diagonally forward with the left leg, keeping your weight mostly on the back leg.

4 Keeping the left knee facing the same way as the toes, turn to the right as you rotate the right shoulder out until the right hand faces to the right. At the same time, move the left arm across with the body, rotating the forearm slightly in so that the palm faces backward.

*(continued on next page)*

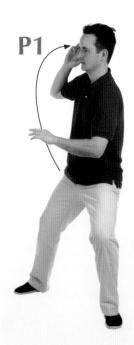

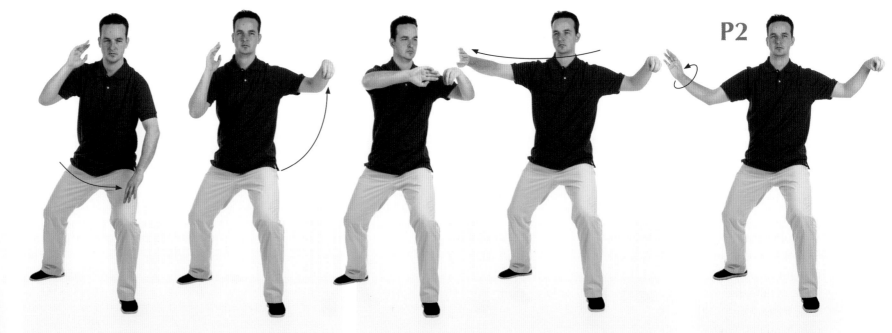

**5** Lower your left hip so that your upper body tilts to the left until it is in line with the back leg. At the same time, raise the right hand up and forward behind your neck, sink the left elbow above the left knee, and lower the left forearm a little, rotating it so that the palm faces down (**P1**; page 76).

**6** As you rotate your body to the left, lower the left hand down. When the hand, with the palm facing left, passes the left leg, make it into a beak. Continue turning the body, but start straightening it as you start pushing your hips forward under your shoulders. Continue raising the left hand (in a beak) up to shoulder level; at the same time, move the right elbow down, slipping the right hand from behind the neck to just in front of it as the body straightens. The right forearm ends in a vertical position.

**7** Turn slightly left as you push the right hand toward the left hand and rotate your right arm out so that your elbow comes up to shoulder level. Turn right as you move the right hand horizontally to the right side. End facing slightly to the right with both arms symmetrical (except for the hands).

**8** Turn your body forward as you relax the hips (as if you are sitting down), and roll the shoulders back and down to relax the arms and sink the elbows. Feel the body sinking to the *dantian* (**P2**).

# 8: Brush Knee 1

> **AT A GLANCE:**
>
> Scoop your arms down, inward, and up as you sink backward into the left Cat Stance and press the arms down.

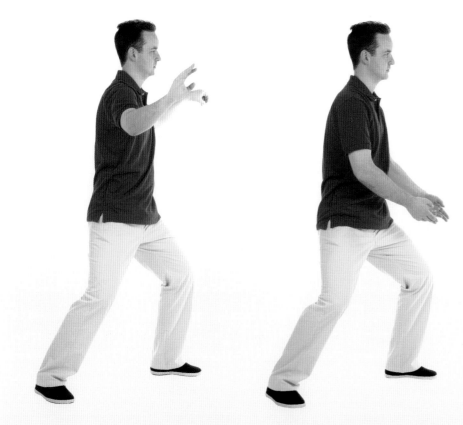

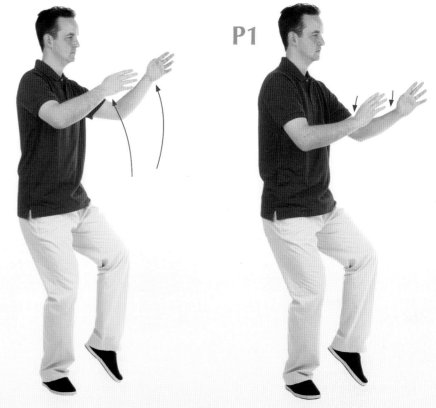

P1

**1** Start in the last posture of the previous movement. Then sink into the front leg as you slowly lower your hands down and in toward the front knee. At the same time, rotate the arms in so that the palms end facing up.

**2** Transfer your weight to the back leg and bring the front foot back into the left Cat Stance as you slowly raise your hands up to shoulder level, and turn the palms to face each other. Relax the hips and arms and sink the elbows. Feel the body sinking to the *dantian* (**P1**; page 77).

# 9: Three Steps Forward 1

### AT A GLANCE:

- Circle both arms—down, right, and up.

- Step forward with the left foot as you push forward with the left hand.

- Step forward with the right foot as you push forward with the right hand.

- Step forward with the left foot as you push forward with the left hand.

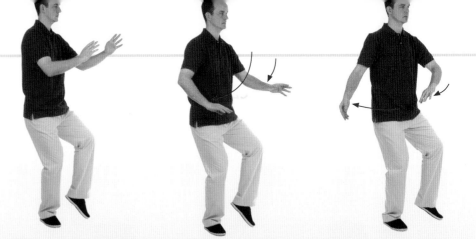

**1** Start in the last posture of the previous movement. Lower both arms and start circling them back and up as you rotate the right arm in (opening the right shoulder). The left hand ends in front of the right shoulder, palm down; the right hand is to the side with the palm facing up.

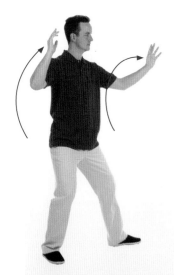

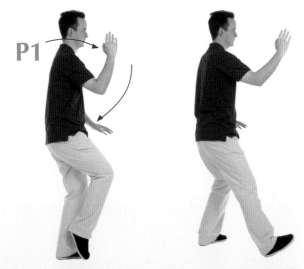

P1

**2** Continue circling the arms and step diagonally forward with the left leg, placing only the heel on the floor as you push the edge of the left hand forward and raise the right hand up.

**3** Continue to circle the arms and transfer your weight to the left leg as you move the right hand past the right ear and the left hand a little forward and downward. Bring the right foot next to the left ankle as you pull the left hand toward the left hip (**P1**; page 77). Step diagonally forward, placing just the heel on the floor as you push the edge of the right hand forward above the right foot and pull the left hand back to the left hip.

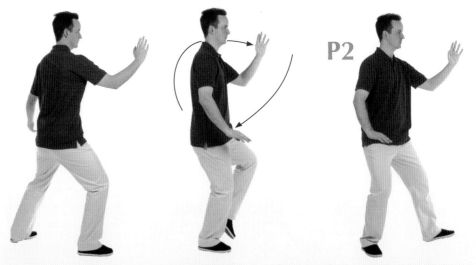

P2

**4** Transfer about 60 percent of your weight forward to the right leg as you rotate the left shoulder out until the left hand faces nearly to the left. Raise the left hand up and forward behind the neck in a circular motion as you transfer all your weight forward, and bring the left foot by the right ankle and move the right hand forward, down, and back to the right hip, with the palm facing down. Step diagonally forward with the left leg, placing only the heel on the floor as you push the edge of the left hand forward and press the right hand a little backward. Immediately slide the left heel a little farther forward as you separate the hands more by pushing the left hand forward and pressing the right hand back (**P2**).

**AT A GLANCE:**

• Turn right and tilt to the left by sinking into the left hip.

• Turn left as you sweep your left hand in front of the left knee and turn it into a beak and raise it to shoulder level. At the same time, move your right hand past your neck and sweep it horizontally left to right.

## Move Sideways 2

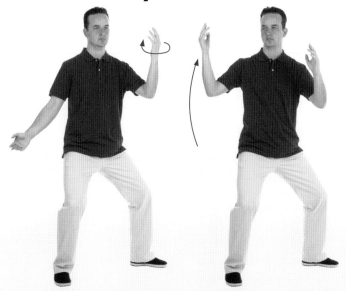 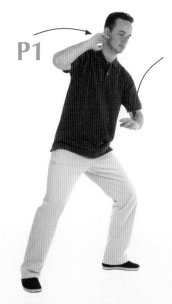 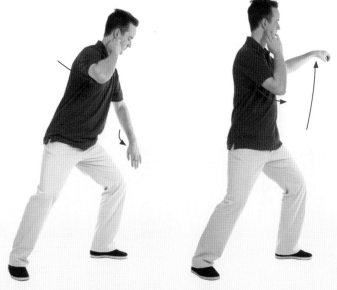

1 Start in the last posture of the previous movement. Keeping the left knee facing the same way as the toes, slowly turn to the right as you rotate the right shoulder out until the right hand faces to the right. At the same time, move the left arm across with the body, rotating the forearm slightly in so that the palm faces backward.

2 Lower your left hip so that your upper body tilts to the left until it is in line with the back leg. At the same time, raise the right hand up and forward behind your neck, sink the left elbow above the left knee, and lower the left forearm a little, rotating it so that the palm faces down (**P1**; page 76).

3 As you rotate your body to the left, lower the left hand down, and when the hand, with the palm facing left, passes the left leg, make it into a beak. Continue turning the body, but start straightening it as you start pushing your hips forward under your shoulders. Continue raising the left hand (in a beak) up to shoulder level; at the same time, move the right elbow down, slipping the right hand from behind the neck to just in front of it as the body straightens. The right forearm ends in a vertical position.

*(continued on next page)*

## Move Sideways 2—continued

## Brush Knee 2

> **AT A GLANCE:**
>
> • Scoop your arms down, inward, and up as you sink backward into the left Cat Stance and press the arms down. (Note that Brush Knee 1 and 2 are identical.)

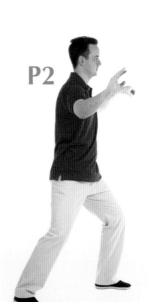

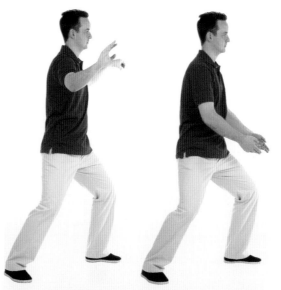

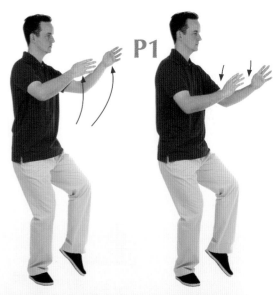

**4** Turn slightly left as you push the right hand toward the left hand and rotate your right arm out so that your elbow comes up to shoulder level. Turn right as you move the right hand horizontally to the right side. End facing slightly to the right with both arms symmetrical (except for the hands).

**5** Turn your body forward as you relax the hips (as if you are sitting down), and roll the shoulders back and down to relax the arms and sink the elbows. Feel the body sinking to the *dantian* (**P2**).

**1** Start in the last posture of the previous movement. Then sink into the front leg as you slowly lower your hands down and in toward the front knee. At the same time, rotate the arms in so that the palms end facing up.

**2** Transfer your weight to the back leg and bring the front foot back into the left Cat Stance as you slowly raise your hands up to shoulder level and turn the palms to face each other. Relax the hips and arms and sink the elbows. Feel the body sinking to the *dantian* (**P1**; page 77).

# 12: Three Steps Forward 2

### AT A GLANCE:

- Circle both arms—down, right, and up.

- Step forward with the left foot as you push forward with the left hand.

- Step forward with the right foot as you push forward with the right hand.

- Step forward with the left foot as you cross the left hand over the right one.

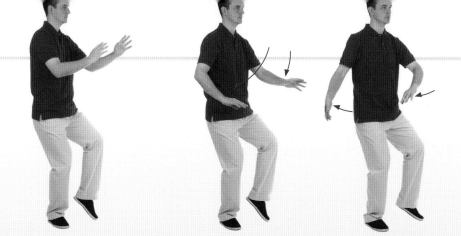

**1** Start in the last posture of the previous movement. Lower both arms and start circling them back and up as you rotate the right arm in (opening the right shoulder). The left hand ends in front of the right shoulder, palm down; the right hand is to the side with the palm facing up.

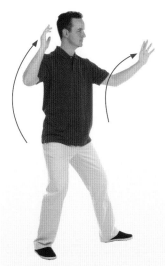

**2** Continue to circle the arms, then step diagonally forward with the left leg, placing only the heel on the floor as you push the edge of the left hand forward and raise the right hand up behind the neck.

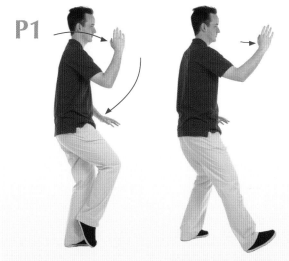

P1

**3** Still circling the arms, transfer your weight to the left leg as you move the left hand a little forward and down and the right hand a little forward, next to the right ear. Bring the right foot next to the left ankle as you pull the left hand toward the left hip (**P1**; page 77). Step diagonally forward, placing just the heel on the floor as you push the edge of the right hand forward above the right foot and pull the left hand back to the left hip.

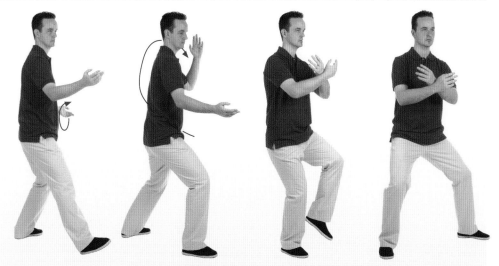

**4** Transfer about 60 percent of your weight forward to the right leg as you rotate the left shoulder out until your left hand faces nearly to the left. Raise your left hand up and forward behind your neck in a circular motion as you transfer all the weight forward, and bring the left foot by the right ankle and move the right hand slightly down. Step diagonally forward with the left leg, placing the foot on the floor as you bring the left arm forward and place the left wrist over the right wrist. End with your body facing the hands, and the palms facing your body.

# 13: Concealed Punch

**AT A GLANCE:**

- Transfer your weight to the left, then to the right, as you turn your body left and right to wind the arms in a circular motion.

- Punch your right fist forward.

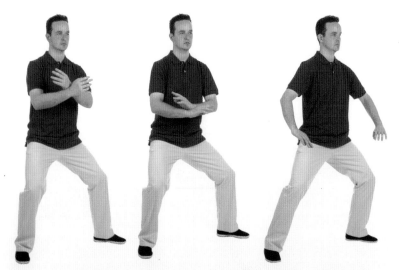
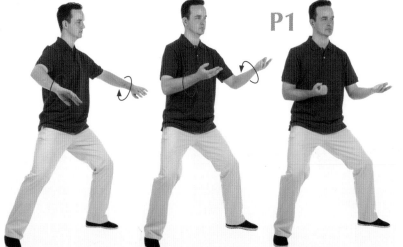
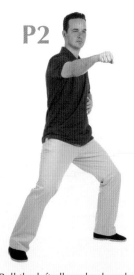

1 Start in the last posture of the previous movement. Sink into the right leg as you slowly lower both arms and turn the hands palms down. Transfer 60 percent of your weight to the left leg as you turn the body left by sinking into the left hip. Open the arms so the hands end up outside the knees, fingers facing in and slightly forward.

2 Transfer 60 percent of your weight to the right leg as you turn to the right and sink into the right hip. At the same time, circle the arms out, up, in, and down while turning both arms in. Your arms end up by your sides with the forearms parallel and pointing in the same direction as the right foot, palms facing up and the right hand closed in a loose fist. The left hand is about 10 inches (25 cm) in front of the right fist (**P1**; page 78).

3 Pull the left elbow back and use a sudden leftward rotation of the hips as you punch the right fist forward. Both your arms rotate outward—the left hand ends touching the left lower ribs with the palm, and the right fist ends up palm down. Don't straighten the right arm fully, and don't use any muscular effort in your arms. As a result of the body turning, about 60 percent of your weight should end on the left leg (**P2**).

# 14: Jin Gang Pounds Mortar 3

**AT A GLANCE:**

- Raise the left hand up to the right forearm as you circle your arms clockwise in a full circle.

- Step with the right leg into a Cat Stance as you pierce the right fingers forward.

- Slam the right fist into the left palm as you stomp the right leg down.

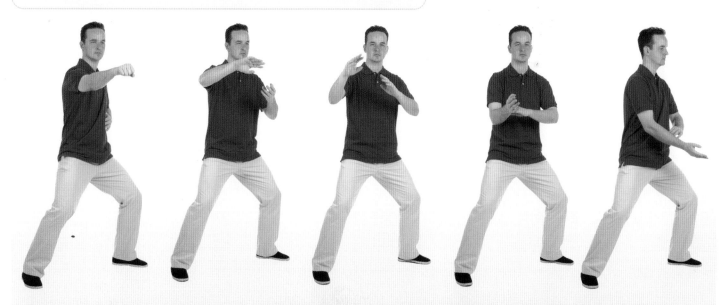 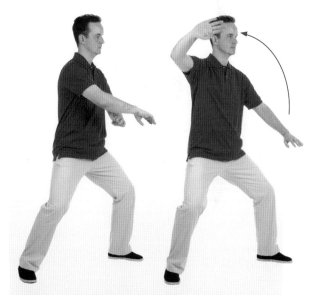

**1** Start in the last posture of the previous movement. Open your right hand as you turn to the right, bringing your arm slightly backward. Use the motion of the body to bring your left hand forward in front of the abdomen. Circle your arms clockwise, moving the right hand as if it is stroking a beach ball and circling the left hand opposite and about twice as fast so that it catches up with the right hand. When the left fingers touch the right forearm, move them together toward the inside of the left knee, the edge of the right hand facing the knee. Throughout this move, the weight hardly changes. When the right hand moves right, sink into the right leg, then sink into the left leg again.

**2** Rotate the right arm out, keeping the left fingers in contact with it. Then transfer 60 percent of your weight to the right leg as you open both arms, pushing the left arm down past the left foot and the right arm opposite it, to the right top corner. End with the right palm facing out and fingers pointing forward.

*(continued on next page)*

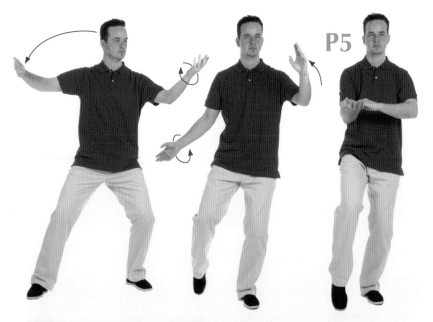

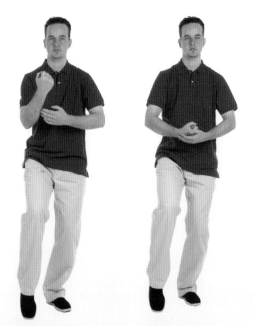

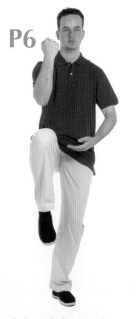

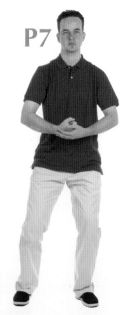

**3** Turn the body and the left foot right as you turn the left hand palm up. Transfer the weight to the left leg as you raise the left hand up to the right and then down.

At the same time, circle the right foot and hand back, in, and forward, turning the right hand palm up. As you start lowering your left arm, step forward with your right leg into the right Cat Stance and move your right arm forward, with the elbow passing close to the body, until the right inside forearm touches the fingers of your descending left hand. The right palm is up and the fingers point forward; the left arm is in the same position from which you just started (**P5**; page 72). When moving forward, the right arm and leg move as one.

**4** Rotate the left palm up as you make a loose fist with your right hand and place it in the left palm. Throughout this move, keep the fingers of the left hand in touch with the right forearm and pivot the right forearm around this point—so that as you raise the right hand up, the elbow goes down; as you move the right hand back toward the left hand, the right elbow circles forward.

**5** Lift the right knee and the right fist as one. The right forearm is vertical; the right foot hangs down (**P6**).

**6** Lift the right foot to a horizontal position, then stomp the right foot down as you slam the right fist into the left palm. The right foot should strike the floor flat as the back of the right fist slams into the left palm (**P7**).

# 15: Closing

Closing is considered the last exercise in this 15-exercise Form. The purpose of the Closing movement is twofold—to return to the starting posture and, more importantly, to help maintain the feeling that was created through the practice. Therefore, try to move very slowly, with your mind calm and undisturbed. Practicing the Closing like this will, in time, enable you to carry the feeling, and the resulting benefits, into your everyday life.

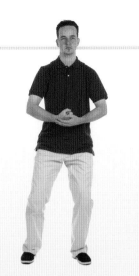 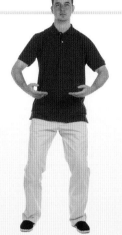 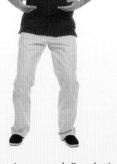 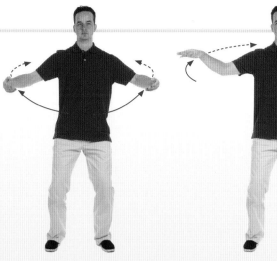 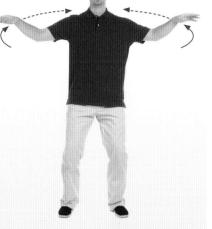

**1** Start in the last posture of the previous exercise as usual. Breathe in as you open your arms and slowly circle them upward, rotating the forearms so that the palms turn facedown as the hands reach shoulder level as shown above right.

## AT A GLANCE:

- Breathe in as you circle your arms up and bring your hands to below the chin.

- Breathe out as you softly press your hands down and move them to your sides, feeling your attention returning to the *dantian*.

- On the next exhalation, bring your feet together.

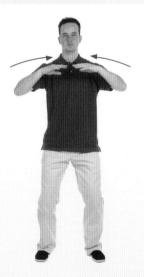 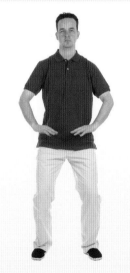 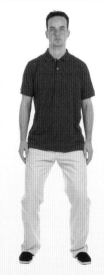 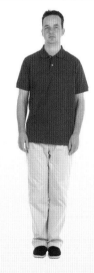

**2** Continue to slowly circle the arms, ending with the hands below your chin and the palms facedown.

**3** Slowly breathe out as you let your hands float down to the *dantian*, relaxing the back and sinking your weight down as you bend your knees.

**4** Keep breathing out as you lower the hands and separate them to the sides of your legs, turning the hands so your palms touch the side of your thighs.

**5** As you slowly straighten the legs, breathe in. You are now in the Basic Stance. Wait until you start breathing out to move your left leg next to the right leg.

# Improving your Tai Chi movement in five stages

Correct movement in the Tai Chi Form is not determined by how precisely you position your arms, legs, and hands in space. The Tai Chi *Classics* say, "Tai Chi should not be pretty." This means that when learning Tai Chi, you should not be trying to make stylish movements. Instead, concentrate on staying relaxed and moving in a natural way, which is the true aim of Tai Chi.

Correctly performed, the Form does look very elegant, but like the beauty of a running cheetah, the beauty of Tai Chi movement is a result of perfect natural balance.

Accurate Tai Chi movement is not something you can achieve overnight. Through repeated practice (over years rather than months) and using sensations and feelings as feedback rather than how you look, you can improve your Tai Chi Form. This long-term goal is best tackled in five stages. At each stage, the movements of your Form will be adjusted as you take up the next challenge.

**Stage 1:** Learn the Form exercise by exercise, and each exercise move by move (as explained on page 80), following the instructions in this chapter.

**Stage 2:** When you feel you are ready to try to improve your movements, practice the Form, concentrating on keeping every part of your body balanced at all times.

**Stage 3:** Next focus on whether each individual movement is moving away from or toward your center or *dantian*. When an arm or leg moves away from your center, feel your body lightly expand with a feeling of a soft stretch from the *dantian* to the end of your fingers or toes.

When an arm or leg moves toward your center, no matter how small the move, feel it emptying and the body sinking to the *dantian*. Start sensing a feeling of connection in the body.

**Stage 4:** During the fourth stage, slowly start sensing your body's connection to the ground. When you step, feel your weight sinking through the leg into the ground. When you turn, feel the effect of your turning on your legs and feet.

**Stage 5:** Eventually, you will start to get a sense of the Central Equilibrium discussed on page 69. From there it is just a short step to Peng, the springlike quality of the body.

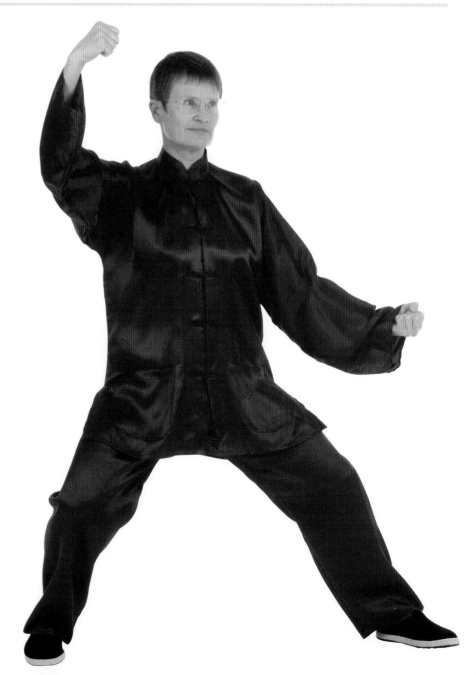

# 8 Practicing the Form

This chapter shows all of the exercises of the Tai Chi Form learned in Chapter 7. Once you have mastered the individual exercises, you can move on to practicing the Form as a single, continuous motion.

*When you practice Tai Chi, stand with your posture balanced like a scale. When you move, your movements should revolve as effortlessly as the turning of a wheel.*

—FROM THE TAI CHI *Classics*

You have learned how to move correctly when doing Tai Chi and have mastered the individual exercises of the Form. Now it is up to you to practice the Form to make it all come together.

The internal connections of the body are like a spider's web, and practicing the Form is like learning how to move your body while retaining the web's integrity and eventually using this web to move your body. You are "tuning" the weblike body structure to move everything together.

Fast moves shake the web, and if the body doesn't move in tune with the web, these movements can disrupt some of the connections. When that happens, it takes time to reestablish the web's taut form. Therefore, practice should be slow and careful at first.

When you practice the Tai Chi Form, think of it as a complex Silk Reeling exercise. Concentrate on trying to feel the body moving through space. At the beginning you may feel only a vague sensation of transferring your weight. As your awareness grows, focus on more details. Eventually, after continued practice of Tai Chi, your movement and awareness will merge together.

## The Form will change

When practicing the Form, do not treat it as a series of fixed-shape movements that you need to perfect. The shape of the individual moves, the timing, and other aspects will change as your strength, flexibility, coordination, and awareness improve. Put your effort into understanding the movement rather than "polishing" the movement.

If you experience difficulties with any of the individual exercises, go back and review the detailed instructions in Chapter 7. Remember that regular practice of Silk Reeling (see pages 53–66) and Zhan Zhuang (see pages 21 and 22) will help you master the Tai Chi Form.

*When one part of the body moves, there is no part that does not move. When one part of the body is still, there is no part that is not still.*

—FROM THE TAI CHI *Classics*

108

# The Form

The Form is shown here as a continuous movement. It should take three to five minutes to perform once all the exercises are flowing together properly one after the other. When starting to practice the Form, keep in mind that the aim is not to try to make Tai Chi look pretty. It does look graceful when practiced correctly, but this comes from observing all the things you have learned about how to move in a balanced, relaxed, natural way.

Remember also to let your head float up and your weight sink down while moving, to always keep a round space under both armpits so that the elbows do not touch the body, and to always point your knees in the same direction as your feet.

Now that you know all the individual exercises, flow them together by following the pictures that start below and continue through page 117.

## Starting the Form

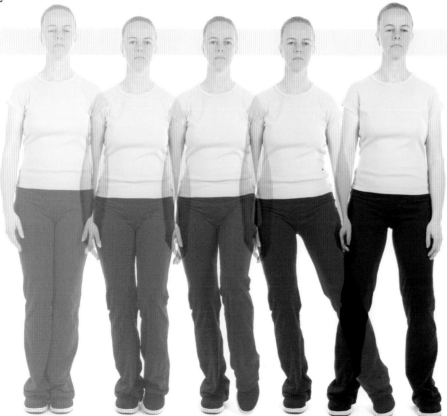

**THE KEY EXERCISES**

The Form in this chapter consists of the same 15 movements you learned in detail in Chapter 7:

 1  Jin Gang Pounds Mortar 1 (see page 84)
 2  Lazy Tying Coat (see page 87)
 3  Six Sealings Four Closings (see page 89)
 4  Single Whip (see page 90)
 5  Jin Gang Pounds Mortar 2 (see page 91)
 6  White Crane Spreads Its Wings (see page 93)
 7  Move Sideways 1 (see page 95)
 8  Brush Knee 1 (see page 97)
 9  Three Steps Forward 1 (see page 98)
10  Move Sideways 2 (see page 99)
11  Brush Knee 2 (see page 100)
12  Three Steps Forward 2 (see page 101)
13  Concealed Punch (see page 102)
14  Jin Gang Pounds Mortar 3 (see page 103)
15  Closing (see page 105)

*Like the beauty of a running cheetah, the beauty of Tai Chi is a result of perfect natural balance.*

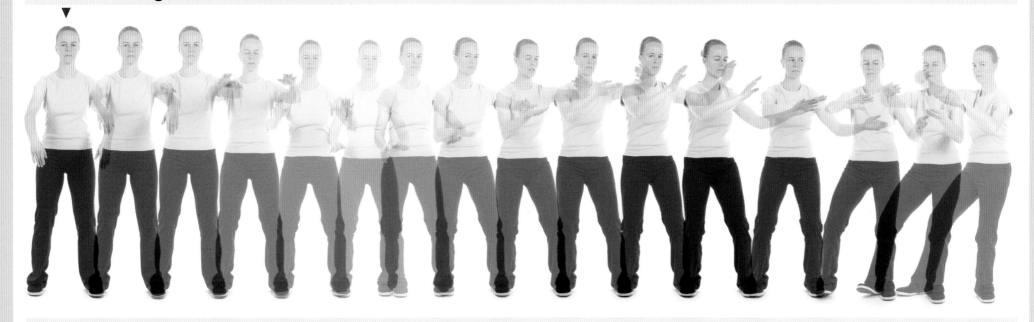

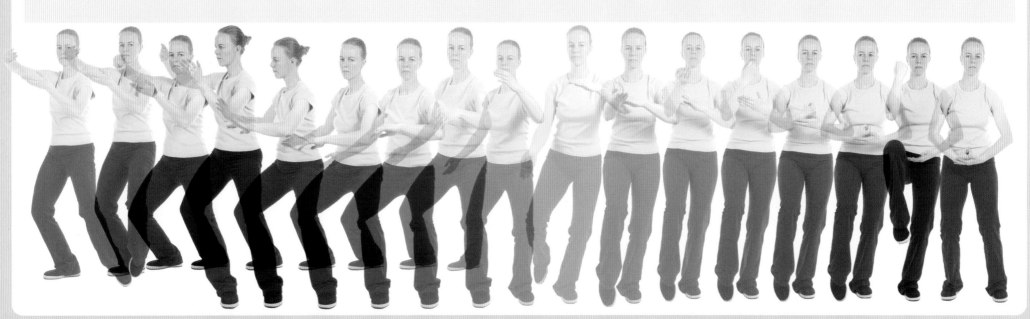

110

## 2: Lazy Tying Coat

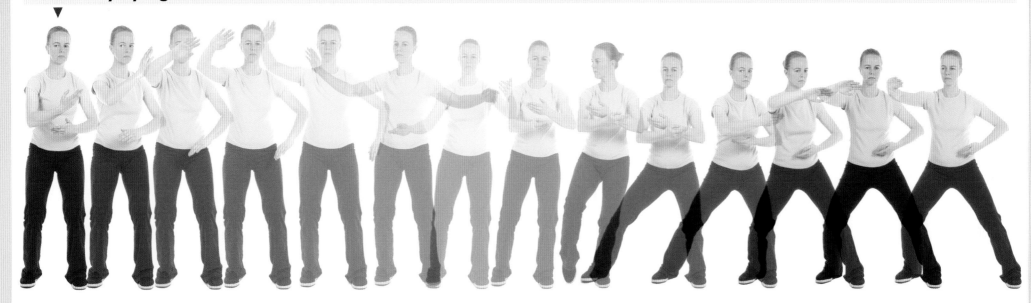

## 3: Six Sealings Four Closings

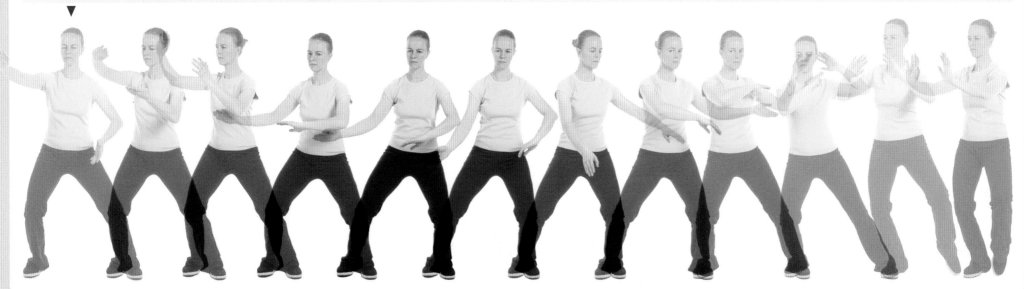

## 4: Single Whip

## 5: Jin Gang Pounds Mortar 2

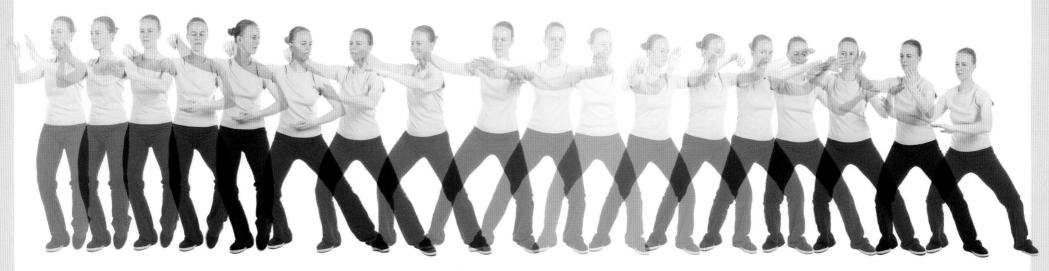

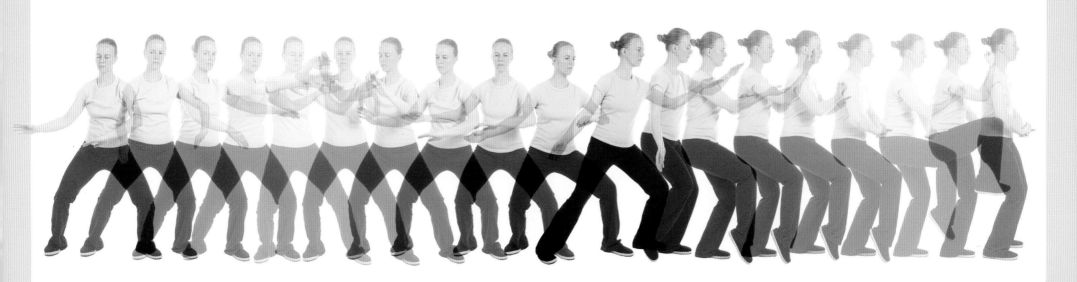

▼                                                          ▼

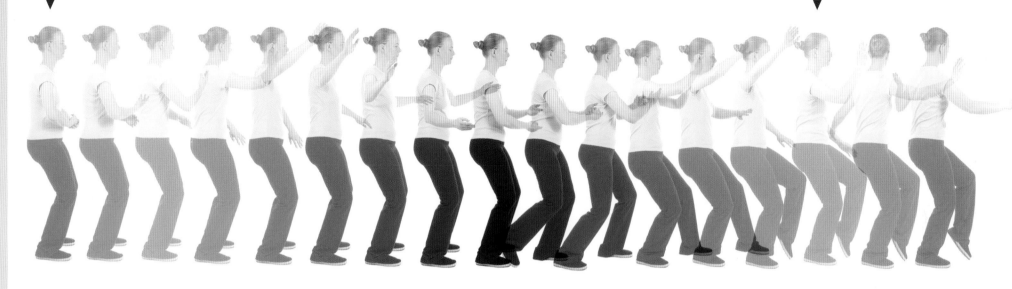

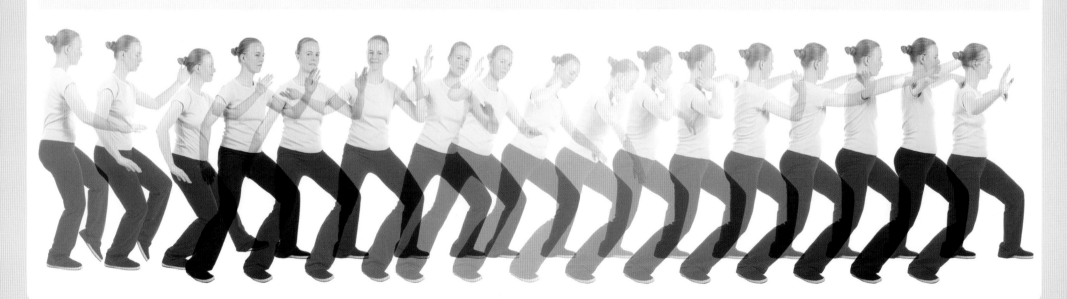

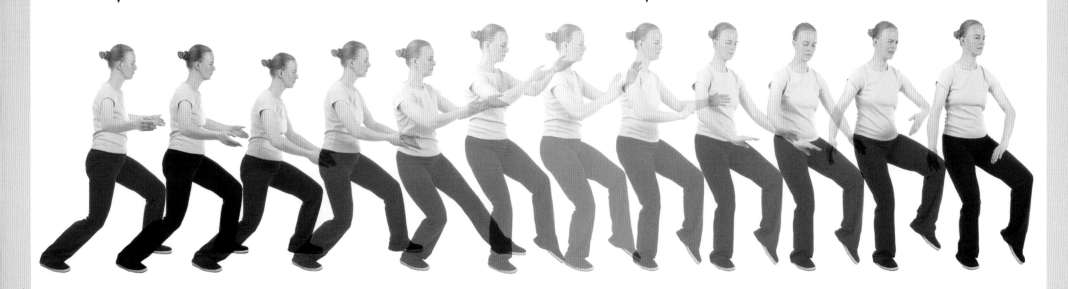

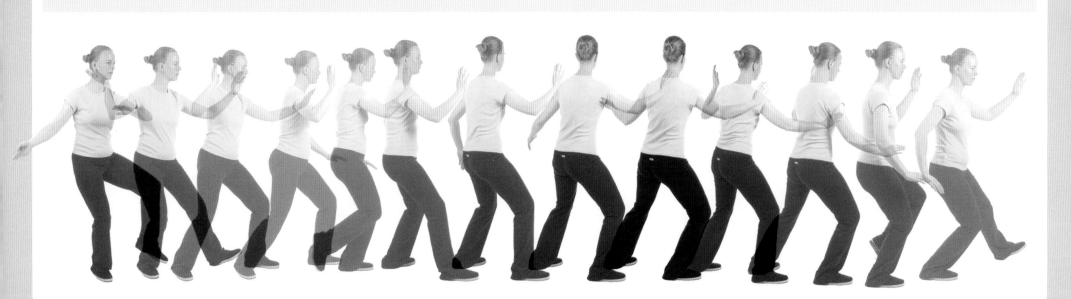

## 10: Move Sideways 2

▼

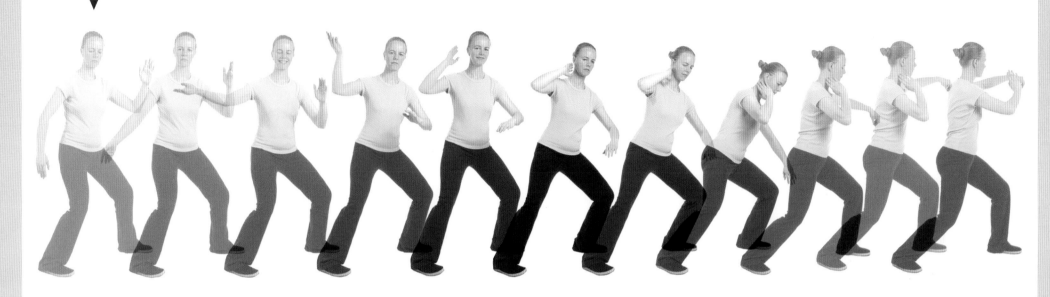

## 11: Brush Knee 2

▼

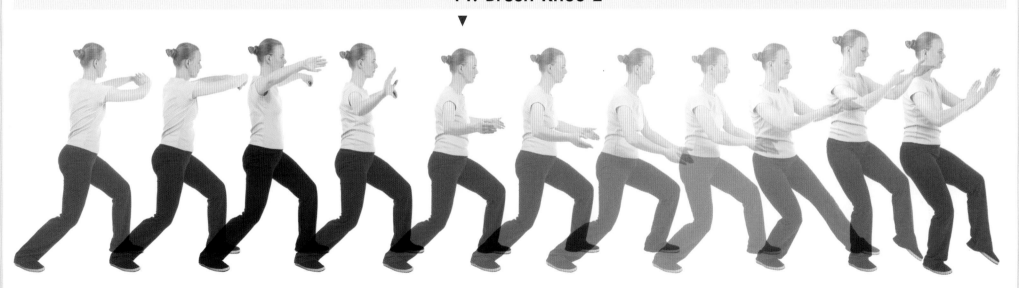

## 12: Three Steps Forward 2

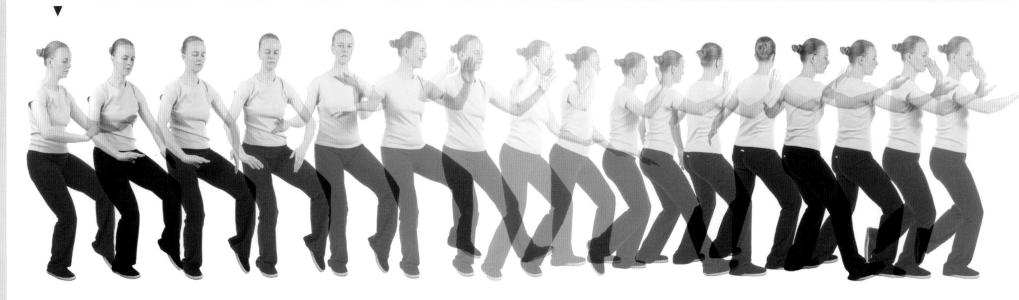

## 13: Concealed Punch

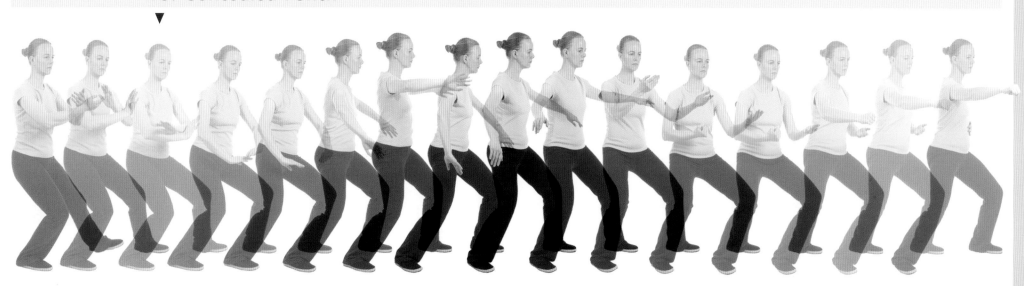

## 14: Jin Gang Pounds Mortar 3

▼

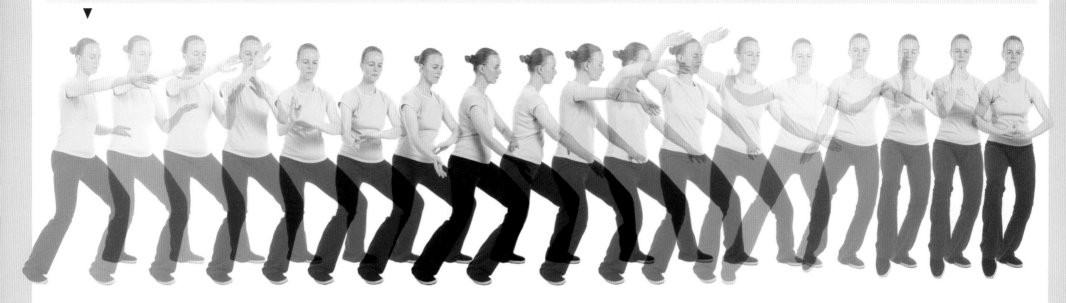

## 15: Closing

▼

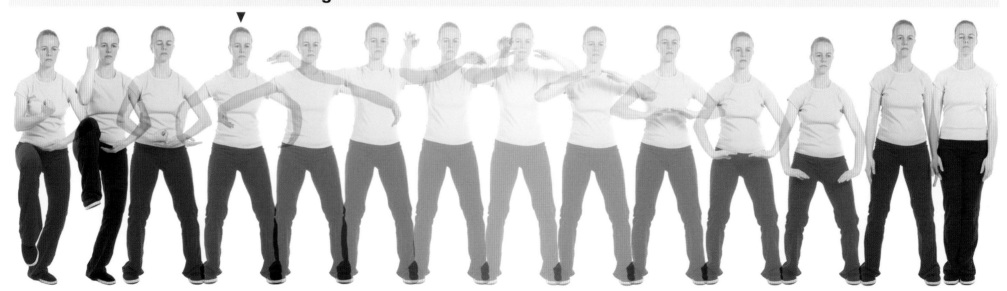

# Practicing in high, middle, and low positions

The way you perform Tai Chi Form movements will change as you continue to practice. But there are some changes to the Form you should make in order to progress. These changes concern the height of your stances.

The Form can be practiced in different heights. Generally, we speak of high, middle, and low positions. Each height has its benefits. The postures in the Form and the various exercises in this book are shown in the high to middle positions. You should learn the Form in the high position and start practicing at this height.

As your body strengthens, start lowering your stances. Do not rush this process; your muscles strengthen faster than the tendons, so allow sufficient time (say, twice or three times as long) before going lower.

When you are comfortable in the low stances, you can change into higher stances again. You want to be able to move in a natural high stance, so that's what you need to practice.

## High position

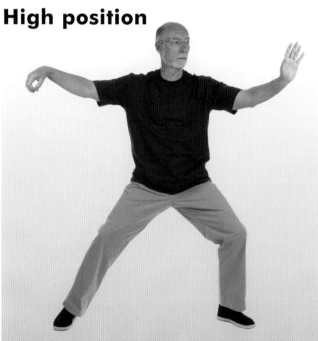

Start practicing the Form in high position. This makes it easier to align the body properly and to relax. Going low too soon results in increased tension due to weakness in deep muscles, especially around the hips; having big muscles from weight training is no help in this regard. The high position is better for aligning the "flow" within the body, especially in hips (*kua*), knees, and ankles.

## Middle position

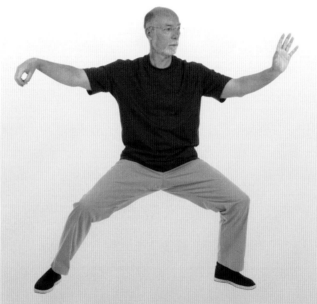

As your body strengthens, lower the stances in your Form to the middle position. Practicing at this height will strengthen your body more, enabling you to go even lower.

## Low position

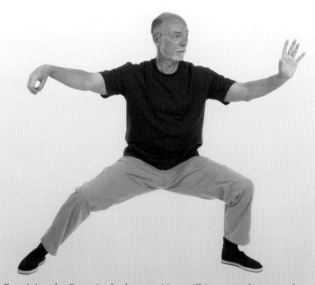

Practicing the Form in the low position will increase the strength in your legs and hips and help you relax the upper body and lower back. It will also help you to sink into the hips. After practicing in low position, go back to high postion to practice agility and sinking.

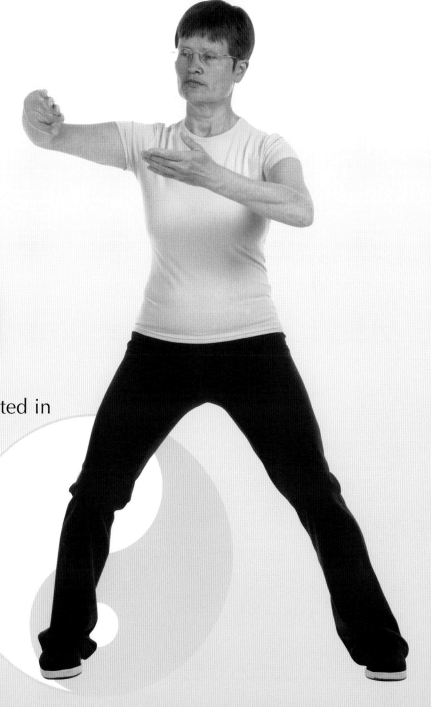

# 9 Using the Mind

This chapter is designed for those interested in taking their Tai Chi regimen to a higher level. It explains Tai Chi theory in more depth and gives exercises for using the mind to improve internal power and strength.

*Use mind, not strength.*

—FROM THE TAI CHI *Classics*

The focus of Tai Chi is to train the mind. In internal martial arts, the role of the mind and how it affects the way we move and exert strength is explained by the Three Internal Harmonies.

According to the Tai Chi theory of the Three Internal Harmonies, the desire (*xin*) to move gives rise to a plan of action or the intent (*yi*) for movement. This intent (*yi*) causes the body to prepare for action by stabilizing itself, which calls up intrinsic energy (*chi*). The actual movement, which is the expression of strength (*li*), is then executed. Since strength (*li*) flows along the route of *chi* and the flow of *chi* precedes it, movement was traditionally thought to be caused by *chi*—hence the saying: "*Chi* leads *li*." The source of *chi* in the human body was said to be the *dantian*, since it is there (deep in the lower abdomen) that the first stabilizing action takes place.

To progress to a higher level with your Tai Chi, you need to improve your ability to support yourself effortlessly against the pull of gravity. This is the key to developing whole-body movement and internal power in Tai Chi. By training this ability to deal with forces other than just gravity, Tai Chi experts are able to perform amazing feats of effortless power.

The difficult part in this type of training is learning how to "control" your body. The way you control your body when balancing is different from the way you control it in "normal" movement.

Staying balanced happens without our conscious involvement, and in Tai Chi theory it is said to be caused by *chi*. (As explained in Chapter 1, in the traditional Chinese view all automatic body processes that happen without our volition, such as blood circulation, digestion and similar, are said to be controlled or caused by *chi*.) The muscular activity of staying balanced also occurs, without our awareness, during consciously led movements.

The following pages in this chapter give guidelines for training your mind to increase internal power. This is called "cultivating the *chi*," and it is an ongoing process that takes several years of Tai Chi practice. It involves increasing the use of tonic or stabilizing muscles (see page 7). The more the tonic muscles are used, the stronger the body absorbs force. Also, the phasic muscles become free to move so you can improve your agility.

## PRESENCE OR ABSENCE OF TENSION

Try holding an object such as a stick or a sword in the positions shown below, and notice the difference in your ability to keep the object vertical when gripping it using force or holding it lightly, feeling the flow of weight along its length. Any tension in the hand and arm will adversely affect your ability to feel the position of the tip in relation to the base.

When practicing advanced Tai Chi with a sword, you will begin to feel the balance of the tip even in nonvertical positions. This is referred to as "extending *chi* to the tip of the sword." In a similar manner, the feeling of balance and control of our own body is affected by presence or absence of tension.

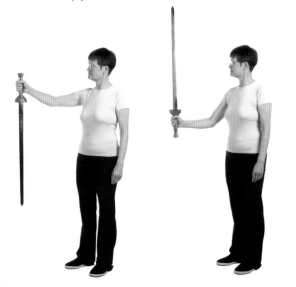

# Using your mind, not your strength

As you learned in Chapter 2 (see pages 21 and 22), the first step in training tonic or stabilizing muscles is the standing practice called Zhan Zhuang. As your Tai Chi practice progresses, you should focus even more attention on standing practice, because it is the best way to train yourself to use the mind over strength.

When practicing Zhan Zhuang, imagine that you are resisting some light force; this tricks the body into going into tonic function. Attempt, at the same time, to consciously relax—this will relax your phasic muscles and enhance the tonic function even more, thus helping to cultivate the *chi*.

Remember that the length of standing practice should be governed by your attention span. When concentration is weakening and other thoughts start to impinge on your mind, make a brief attempt to come back to the practice. If it fails, however, end the training for the day (or the time being). This way, your concentration will gradually improve with the standing in a natural way. The process is quite simple.

As your standing practice improves, gradually you will become aware of areas of the body that you were not aware of before. This will help you to keep your mind focused during the standing practice. Because you have more of the body to observe, you can perform standing practice even longer without getting bored.

So if on your first day of trying Zhan Zhuang you exhaust your observation in five seconds, stop after five seconds. After six months you may be fully occupied and fascinated by observing the changing sensations in your body for as long as five or ten minutes. This is the easiest, and most likely the quickest, route to success—don't ever let standing practice feel boring.

Standing in Zhan Zhuang and watching television is better than sitting and watching television, but it shouldn't be thought of as replacing the standing practice where you fully concentrate on the body.

**Zhan Zhuang Position 1**

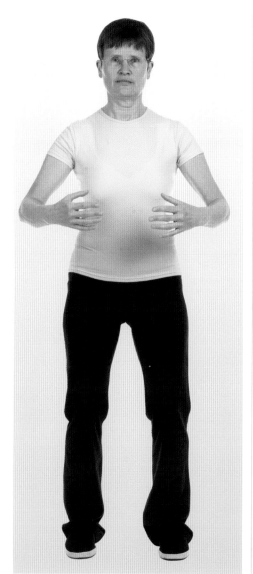

**Zhan Zhuang Position 2**

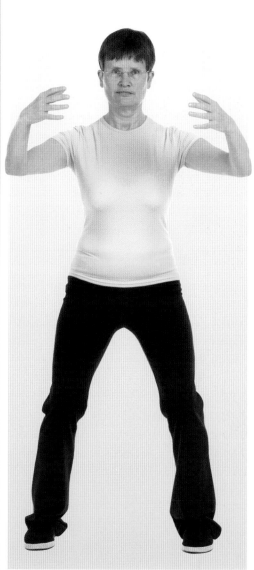

# Internal and external connections

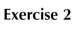

So far you have learned how to hold a soft and relaxed posture. Explained here is how to hold our body when it's being used to do something. For example, if you are pushing a fairly heavy cart up a slope, the force comes from the legs. The upper body and arms just transmit the force to the cart. To transmit the force efficiently, you need to make the connection from the legs to the cart (the connection being the arms and the body) strong enough so that it does not collapse. If the connection is strengthened using stabilizing muscles, this is an internal connection (the stabilizers are usually deeper and there are no signs of muscle tension on the surface of the body). If the connection is strengthened using phasic muscles, this is an external connection. Look at the effect these two types of connections have on the body by trying the two exercises on the right.

These two examples should convince you that using phasic muscles tends to distort your alignment. Also when you compare the two postures, the posture achieved in Exercise 2 feels more balanced.

Stabilizing muscles act in response to forces acting on our body unlike the phasic muscles, whose action is usually predetermined by will. This means that external connections, since they cannot easily adapt to changing circumstances (for example, changing angles), tend to be stiffer than internal ones. As you give up using conscious tension, you will see other differences.

**Exercise 1**

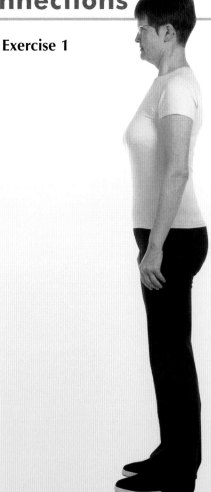

Stand in the Basic Stance. Quickly extend your body as high as you can. Doing it quickly ensures that you use phasic muscles. What probably happens is that you arch your back and can feel tension throughout the body. The places of tension should be fairly easy to locate.

**Exercise 2**

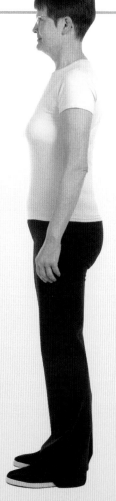

Try it again, this time using stabilizers. Stand in the Basic Stance. Imagine that your head is suspended by a string from above and it is slowly being pulled upward, letting your head slowly float up and feeling it pull the rest of the spine with it. Observe the state of your body, especially your chest and lower back. If you notice tension creeping in anywhere in the body, relax that area and keep slowly expanding upward. What should happen is that your body does not markedly change its shape. There is either no tension felt, or if there is, it is much less pronounced and difficult to locate.

# How to move in Tai Chi

You need to train your Tai Chi movement so that it is a result of an intent-controlled stabilizing system, not a result of consciously controlled movement. This can be achieved by a combination of relaxing your muscles as much as possible, pretending someone or something else is moving you, and using kinesthetic images—for example, moving as if you are submerged in water.

Since you consciously control only the phasic muscles (those responsible for movement), consciously relaxing your muscles means relaxing your phasic muscles. Moving as if your body was moved by something other than yourself will help you relax the phasic muscles even more. After practicing like this a long time, the continuous changing pattern of the stabilizers will by itself carry your movement. Your body will feel as if it's floating without any effort. Moving against imagined light resistance promotes further engagement of stabilizers. This is necessary for development of Central Equilibrium and Peng.

The next stage, for those interested in Tai Chi as a martial art, would be to train the phasic muscles to provide explosive strength (*fajin*) and to learn partner practice (Pushing Hands).

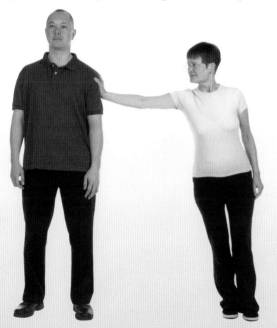

Above, the teacher's arm muscles are relaxed and she is using her arm to balance herself against the student. This demonstrates the way arms should be used in Tai Chi—for example, when pushing or punching. Try balancing with your arm like this to feel the sensations in the arm.

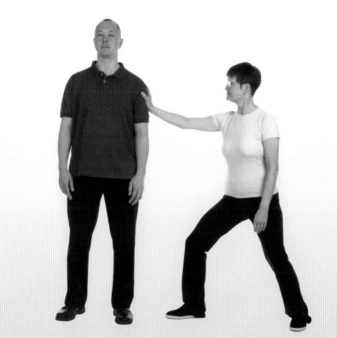

In Tai Chi, you use your arms only to transmit, not to generate strength. Above, the teacher is using the arm in the same way she did for balancing; the arm is aligned and the arm muscles are relaxed. Her strength is generated in the legs and augmented by the torso. If the student moves sideways, she will have no problem redirecting the push toward his center.

## USING FEEDBACK

Any type of learning needs some feedback to help guide the process of learning. In Tai Chi the sensation of using strength is a reliable indication that we are using phasic muscles. But you can also get feedback from other internal sensations or feelings that are more directly related to the use of stabilizers. These sensations are usually vague and often nonexistent to a beginner, and for some of them we do not really have a vocabulary capable of describing them. What you need to do is constantly practice with an attitude of observing what your body does and how it feels.

When practicing, you will eventually become aware of an unbelievable amount of detail in your movement or postures. Some people may feel nothing to start with, but with continuing awareness and practice, the amount will grow.

nce you have practiced the Silk Reeling exercises in Chapter 5 until the movement feels natural and comfortable, you are ready to learn more about *chi* circulation, *dantian* rotation, and whole-body movement.

There is a saying in Tai Chi: "Where the mind goes, *chi* follows." Use this idea to help guide your movement in these advanced Silk Reeling lessons. To the right, *chi* refers to the sensation extending from the *dantian* to some point in the body. For example, *chi* at the elbow means the sensation extending from the *dantian* to the elbow.

Imagine your movement as a flow, progressing through your body in a continuous wave, and follow this wave with your mind as if you were sensing the flow. Don't worry if you can't sense anything; as your awareness increases, you will start feeling a number of sensations and they will change.

After you can comfortably follow the flow of *chi*, gradually shift the mental focus from treating *chi* as a consequence of the movement and start treating it as a cause of the movement. Feel your mind directing the sensation flow and feel the flow affect your body to make the movement happen.

After a lot more practice it will all start making sense!

## Single-Hand Silk Reeling

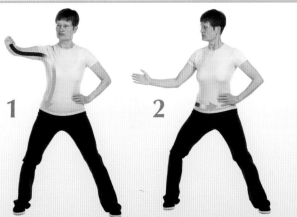 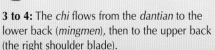

**1 (first position):** The *chi* is at the fingertips of the right hand.
**1 to 2:** The *chi* flows from the fingertips through the elbow to the right side of the waist.
**2 to 3:** The *chi* flows from the right side of the waist along the lower abdomen to the *dantian*.

**3 to 4:** The *chi* flows from the *dantian* to the lower back (*mingmen*), then to the upper back (the right shoulder blade).
**4 to 1:** The *chi* flows from the upper back, through the shoulder and elbow, to the right hand (fingertips).

The *chi* that flows from the fingertips to the *dantian* (**1** to **3**) is toward the center and is called *Yin chi*. The *chi* that flows from the *dantian* to the fingertips (**3** to **4** to **1**) is away from the center and is called *Yang chi*.

## Reverse Single-Hand Silk Reeling

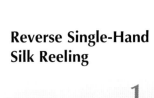 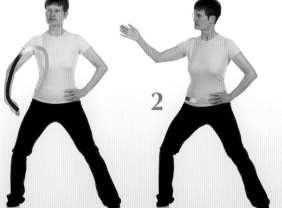 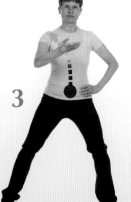 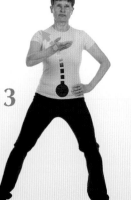 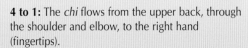

**1 (first position):** The *chi* is at the fingertips of the right hand.
**1 to 2:** The *chi* flows from the fingertips through the elbow to the right side of the waist.

**2 to 3:** The *chi* flows from the right side of the waist along the lower abdomen to the *dantian*.
**3 to 4:** The *chi* flows from the *dantian* to the lower back (*mingmen*), then to the upper back (the right shoulder blade).

**4 to 1:** The *chi* flows from the upper back, through the shoulder and elbow, to the right hand (fingertips).

# *Dantian* to the hands—Double-Hand Silk Reeling

To practice advanced Double-Hand Silk Reeling, combine the advanced Single-Hand Silk Reeling and Reverse Single-Hand Silk Reeling that you learned on the previous page. If you find the combined images difficult to follow, practice the single-hand versions until the accompanying sensations become more or less automatic.

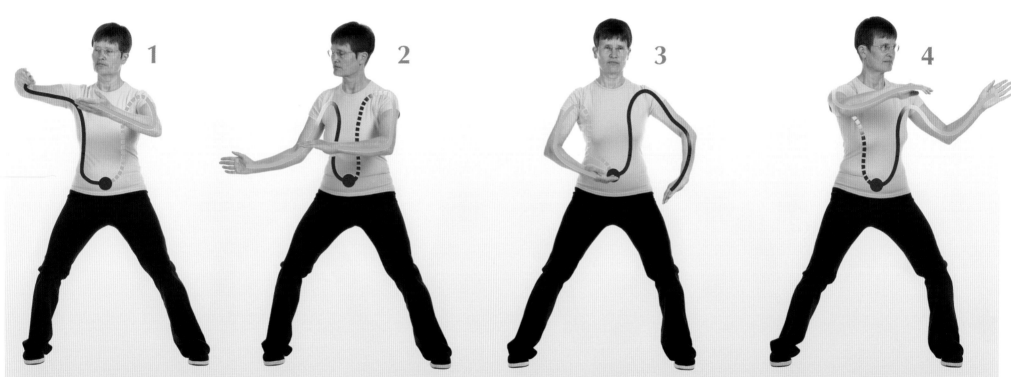

**1 (first position)—right side:** The *chi* is at the fingertips of your right hand. **Left side:** The *chi* is at the *dantian*.
**1 to 2—right side:** The *chi* flows from the fingertips through the elbow to the right side of the waist. **Left side:** The *chi* flows from the *dantian* to the lower back (*mingmen*), then to the upper back (the left shoulder blade).

**2 to 3—right side:** The *chi* flows from the right side of the waist, along the lower abdomen to the *dantian*. **Left side:** The *chi* flows from the upper back, through the shoulder and elbow, to the left hand (fingertips).
**3 to 4—right side:** The *chi* flows from the *dantian* to the lower back (*mingmen*), then to the upper back (the right shoulder blade).

**Left side:** The *chi* flows from the fingertips, through the elbow, to the left side of the waist.

**4 to 1—right side:** The *chi* flows from the upper back, through the shoulder and elbow, to the right hand (fingertips). **Left side:** The *chi* flows from the left side of the waist along the lower abdomen to the *dantian*.

# Dantian rotation—Single-Hand Silk Reeling

In whole-body movement in Tai Chi, all parts of the body move and the movement is centered and directed from the *dantian*. The *dantian*, together with the legs, is the main engine that drives the movement.

Chapter 5 introduced you to the use of the *dantian* in Tai Chi Silk Reeling, and to take your Tai Chi to a more advanced level, you need to further train how to use it as the engine to your movement. The exercise below will help you with this training. It does not give detailed instructions on exactly how to move the *dantian*; this is something you will discover through observation and experimentation.

To close or open a *kua* during the exercise, close or open the relevant inguinal crease (the diagonal crease in the groin). Closing a *kua* also involves relaxing the same hip and sinking your weight down through the leg; it is also called "sinking into a *kua*." When one *kua* closes, the opposite *kua* usually opens.

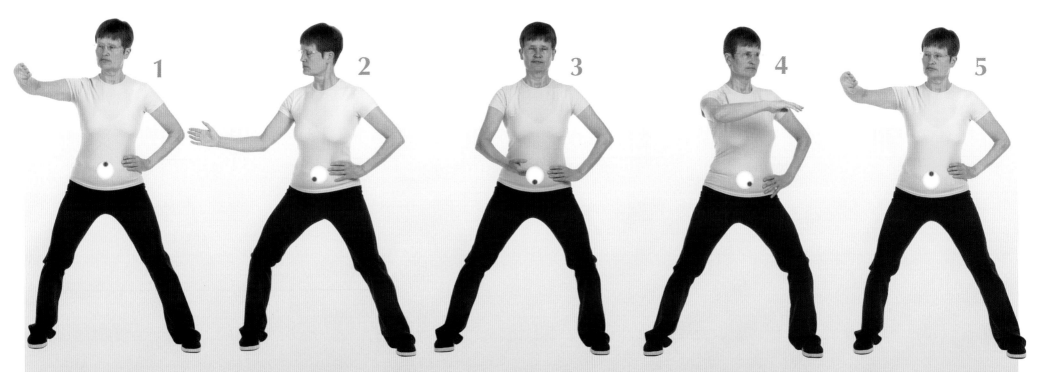

Practice Single-Hand Silk Reeling in the usual way (as in the steps above), while imagining that there is a string connecting your right hand to your navel. As you circle the hand, feel your navel (and hence the *dantian*) being pulled around. Whenever you turn to one side, the *kua* on that side closes and the opposite one opens. As you roll the *dantian*, make sure the lower back doesn't tighten. After practicing with the right hand, do the same with the left hand.

Feel the *dantian* as a ball rolling around in your abdomen as above. Try to sense the rotation rather than force it. This exercise will take time; be patient and do not hurry. Little by little, day by day, your awareness of the rotation will grow and your movement will adapt to the new understanding.

When you can feel the *dantian* rolling freely like a ball, start treating the *dantian* as the driving force and feel your body follow the *dantian*'s

rotation. At first, let the body's movement lag slightly behind the *dantian* so that it looks like the body is pulled by the *dantian*. Gradually, start shortening this lag until the *dantian* and the body move together.

# *Dantian* to the legs—Single-Hand Silk Reeling

On pages 124 and 125 you explored spirals in your upper body. There should be a similar flow in the lower body. This flow should be the same for all Silk Reeling exercises.

There is one difference between the spirals in the arms and the legs. The *dantian* to the hand-body segment forms what is called an open kinetic chain (that means that one end, the *dantian*, is fixed, and the other end, the hand, is free to move). However, the *dantian* to the foot-body segment forms what is called a closed kinetic chain (both ends are fixed), so the force or movement is felt in the whole leg at once. This gives a choice when you are transferring your weight from one leg to another; think of it as pushing up from the foot, or pushing down from the *dantian* to the same foot. The effect is the same, but if you train to push from the *dantian* to the ground, your movement will be more balanced and coordinated. Experiment with both views to help you increase your awareness of the legs-*dantian* connection.

Use this exercise to train the use of the *dantian*.

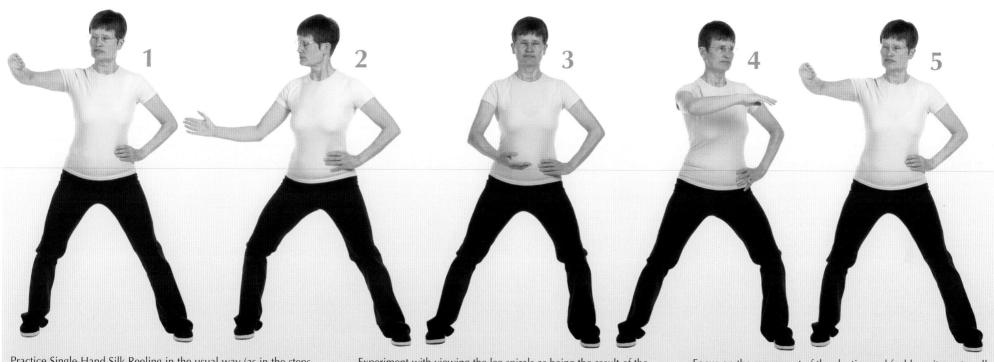

Practice Single-Hand Silk Reeling in the usual way (as in the steps above). When transferring weight from leg to leg, keep the knees fixed to point in the same direction as the toes. Rotation of the *dantian* produces a twisting motion in the legs. After a time, this twisting motion will become independent of the *dantian* rotation and will feel like spirals flowing freely through the legs. Try to sense the spirals in the legs; do not try to create them.

Experiment with viewing the leg spirals as being the result of the *dantian* rotation and then again as the cause of the *dantian* rotation. Eventually, the leg spirals and the *dantian* rotation merge into one motion.

You now have all the elements of complete Silk Reeling motion. With more practice the spirals in the upper and lower body will integrate via the *dantian* rotation into a whole-body motion.

Focus on the movement of the *dantian* and feel how it creates all other spirals; the spirals in turn will move the rest of the body. Eventually, you will be able to feel as if the joints of your body are interconnected cog wheels—you just move the center wheel and the whole body moves in a smooth, coordinated fashion. When you can feel this type of motion in Silk Reeling exercises, you will naturally use it in your Form practice.

# Movement and stillness

According to the Tai Chi *Classics*, in Tai Chi there should be both "movement in stillness" and "stillness in movement." To advance in Tai Chi, you need a good understanding of these two concepts.

## Movement in stillness

When practicing Zhan Zhuang (see pages 21 and 22), you will observe that even when standing still, your body constantly makes small adjustments to its position. The only way you can prevent movement and keep parts of your body still would be to tense your muscles.

If you can't detect movement when doing standing practice, it might be because your body is tense or that the movement is so small you are not aware of it. To make these balancing adjustments more obvious, stand on one leg for a while and observe your body. These small adjustments can be used as an indication of how relaxed you are.

Go through the vertical axis of your body and see if you can make your body balance along its whole length. The more places where you can induce this balancing action, the more relaxed and more balanced you become, and the adjusting movements

grow smaller. So the "movement in stillness" is a direct consequence of not using phasic muscles to support your posture, since you can only tense phasic muscles.

## Stillness in movement

In "How to move in Tai Chi" on page 123 you have seen that eliminating the use of phasic muscles from movement results in a floating sensation with no feeling of effort. There is also a sense that you have to continuously provide an "intent to move" to keep the movement going—unlike in a phasic-led movement, which needs an intent only at the beginning.

If you withdraw that intent, the movement will come to a stop. There is no sense of active movement; the body feels as if it is resting and someone is moving it along. There is a feeling of stillness within movement. This feeling of stillness is further enhanced by the mind's ability to "stretch time" in moments of total concentration. As the scope of your awareness increases, time will seem to slow down while you float effortlessly through space.

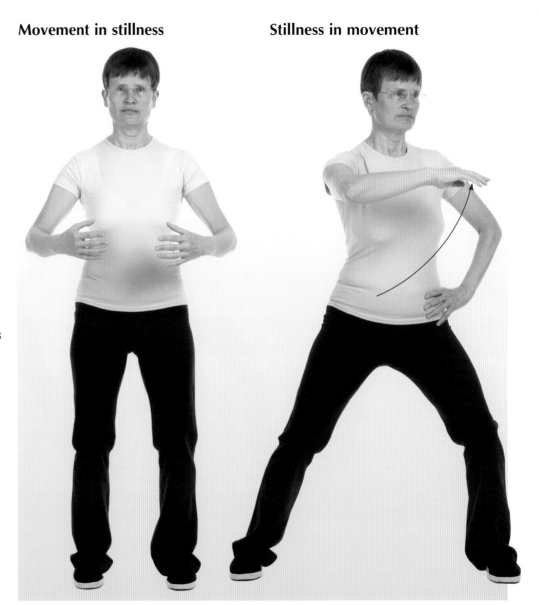

**Movement in stillness**

**Stillness in movement**

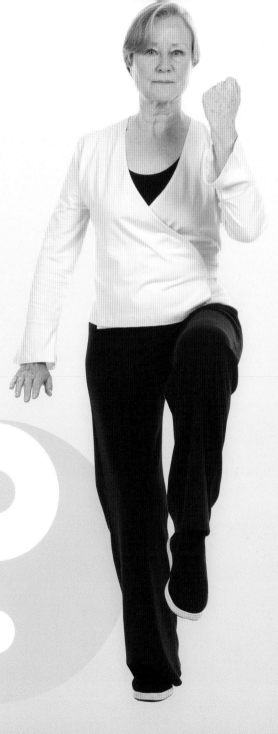

# 10 Tai Chi for Health

Learning Tai Chi well can take a long time, so it is fortunate that practicing Tai Chi will give you the health and the strength to be active long enough to master it!

*The greatest revelation is stillness.*

—FROM *Dao De Jing* BY LAO TZU

After a period of regular practice, you will feel the effects of Tai Chi in your improved physical, mental, and emotional well-being.

On a physical level, if you practice Tai Chi regularly, your body will become stronger and more supple; your movements will gain poise and become more graceful due to improved posture, balance, and coordination.

On a mental level, you will be able to think more clearly and your concentration will be improved.

On an emotional level, you will become more relaxed, tolerant, and generally happier.

## Anyone can practice Tai Chi

Because Tai Chi movement is very slow, anyone can practice this form of exercise. You can even practice Tai Chi into an advanced age. It is not uncommon to see practitioners in their 80s and 90s move with the strength and grace of someone 20 to 30 years younger.

## Eliminates stress

Because the pace of modern life increases continually, our stress levels seem to be increasing, too. Although we need a certain amount of stress to remain healthy, high levels of stress are implicated in a number of undesirable conditions, such as high blood pressure, problems with digestion, and a weakened immune system.

Tai Chi is particularly suited to helping us destress, because correct practice is based on relaxation of the body and mind. The quiet and gentle nature of the exercise helps to overcome stress and its related problems and illnesses. The natural, even, relaxed breathing of Tai Chi also has a calming effect both on the body and the mind.

## Improves mobility

Regular Tai Chi practice, and the Silk Reeling motion in particular, is excellent for the strength and mobility of joints and connective tissue. The combination of soft and relaxed movement with a full range of motion improves the health of the joints.

## Strengthens bones

As a weight-bearing exercise, Tai Chi can also increase bone density and help prevent osteoporosis. This is a real plus for those approaching middle age to help hold off the natural lessening of bone strength.

## Improves heart function

It has been shown in clinical trials that the practice of Tai Chi results in a smoother heart rate and a lower blood pressure. Studies indicate that Tai Chi is clearly more effective than ordinary aerobic exercise.

**Practicing Tai Chi outdoors**
The fact that Tai Chi can be practiced outdoors in peaceful surroundings, increases its ability to relieve stress.

# Posture and health

Because Tai Chi focuses primarily on achieving good posture and balance, it is one of the best exercise systems for reeducating the body to use postural muscles correctly.

It has been recognized recently that good posture plays a very important role in overall health. An estimated 99 percent of adults have poor posture, and this is the cause of most musculoskeletal problems—backaches, neck strains, joint problems, and so on. Poor posture can also cause a number of problems resulting from the compression or distortion of internal organs (due to decreased space in the chest and abdomen), such as respiratory and circulation disorders, and constipation and other gastrointestinal problems. In addition, poor posture can cause rheumatism, arthritis, and even stress.

Our posture is maintained, without our awareness, by muscle reflexes that are learned in childhood. Poor posture can be adopted at any time during our lives, and it is almost inevitable due to the amount of time we spend sitting on chairs, which weakens leg, hip, and back muscles. Prolonged mental stress and holding a fixed posture for a long period of time at school or work can also adversely affect posture. Even sports can be detrimental if they encourage muscular imbalances.

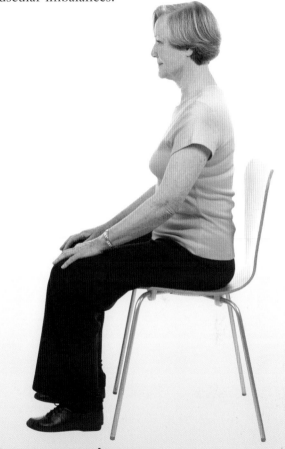

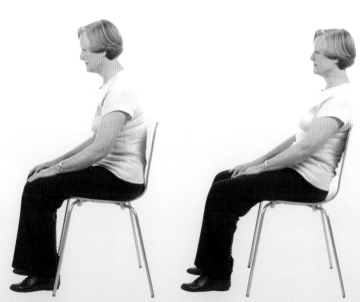

### Weak muscles
These two postures are typical for someone whose postural muscles are either weak or are not being used properly.

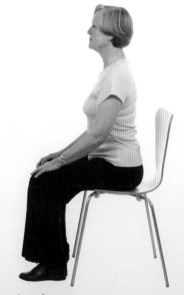

### Strained posture
This posture is the effect of consciously trying to straighten the back. The arched back and tense neck cause strain in the back muscles, which will result in one of the postures on the left being adopted again.

### Correct, natural posture
This is a naturally held correct posture that can be easily achieved through a period of correct Tai Chi practice. The whole body is relaxed. The spine is straight, and both the spine and head are well balanced. The head feels as if it is floating upward.

# Balance and coordination

Balance is increasingly seen as an important player in a healthy lifestyle—especially in the later stages of our lives. Practicing Tai Chi has a very positive impact on the sense of balance and can improve your balance by nearly 50 percent.

Scientific research showed that learning Tai Chi is more effective in improving balance than any other intervention—even more effective than a computer-controlled program of exercises specially designed for improving balance. Balance improvement through Tai Chi has a lasting effect, whereas the effect of static balancing exercises does not seem to last.

Once you have learned the Tai Chi Form, you will see how your coordination improves. Tai Chi coordination is not just the coordination of movement, but also the coordination of the deep postural muscles, of the breathing system, and, ultimately, of the whole body and mind.

When you practice Tai Chi regularly, the process of health improvement takes place gradually by small changes and is mostly unnoticed. One day you wake up and realize that you haven't been ill for a long time, your pains and aches have disappeared, and you always have plenty of energy and enjoy moving and living!

## HOW TAI CHI IMPROVES BALANCE

There are a number of reasons why balance improves through the practice of Tai Chi. Because of the slow rate of movement in Tai Chi, each time you lift a leg, your balance is given a challenge and a workout. Another contribution to improved balance comes from greatly increased leg strength. With Tai Chi, balance improves rapidly as well—improvement in balance is one of the first two things students mention (the other is how well they sleep).

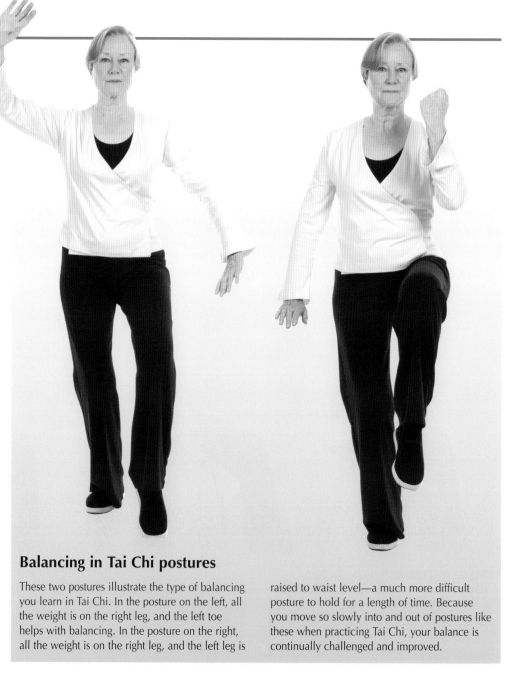

## Balancing in Tai Chi postures

These two postures illustrate the type of balancing you learn in Tai Chi. In the posture on the left, all the weight is on the right leg, and the left toe helps with balancing. In the posture on the right, all the weight is on the right leg, and the left leg is raised to waist level—a much more difficult posture to hold for a length of time. Because you move so slowly into and out of postures like these when practicing Tai Chi, your balance is continually challenged and improved.

# Testing your balance

When you start out, rate your balance with the simple test on this page. You can then test yourself later as your Tai Chi improves.

Follow the steps on the right to take the test. Using a stopwatch or getting someone else to time you, perform the test three times and choose the best time. Find your score in the box below.

If you can balance according to your age or better, congratulations and keep up the good work. If you find that your balance falls far short of your actual age, remember that you can improve your balance with a little bit of Tai Chi practice—and you can keep on improving it. Perform the test after a few weeks of Tai Chi and watch the years fall off!

## BALANCING TEST

| If you can balance for... | You have the balance of a... |
|---|---|
| 2.5 seconds | 60-year-old |
| 3.7 seconds | 50-year-old |
| 7.2 seconds | 40-year-old |
| 15.1 seconds | 30-year-old |
| 22.1 seconds | 20-year-old |

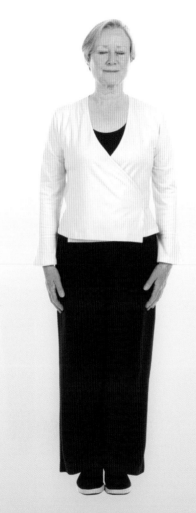

1 Stand with your feet together and your hands at your sides and relax in this position. Close your eyes.

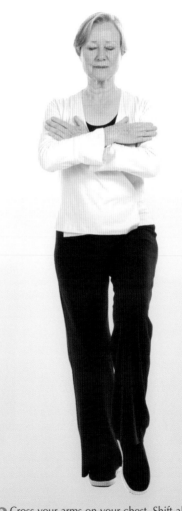

2 Cross your arms on your chest. Shift all your weight onto the right leg and bend the left knee.

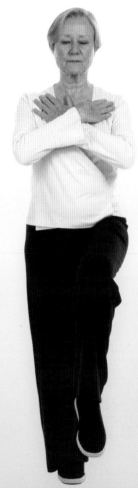

3 Start the count. Lift your left foot off the floor and hold this position as long as you can without moving the supporting foot or letting the raised foot down. Stop the count.

# Simple balancing exercise

It is a good idea to practice balancing exercises on a daily basis. Some of these are simple exercises that can be easily incorporated in your daily life. For example, stand on your toes when you brush your teeth or wait for a kettle to boil. When waiting in a line, feel your body soften and notice the continuous adjustments that happen when you let go of habitual tension.

Eventually, you will start noticing these and similar sensations during normal movement—as you walk, sit down, get up, reach for something. You will be able to stop practicing at a designated time and start practicing at all times!

Here is a simple balancing exercise that you can do on your own or with friends.

## USE THIS MENTAL IMAGE

In step 3, stretch your body upward as if you are pushing something up with your hands.

## Pushing Against the Sky

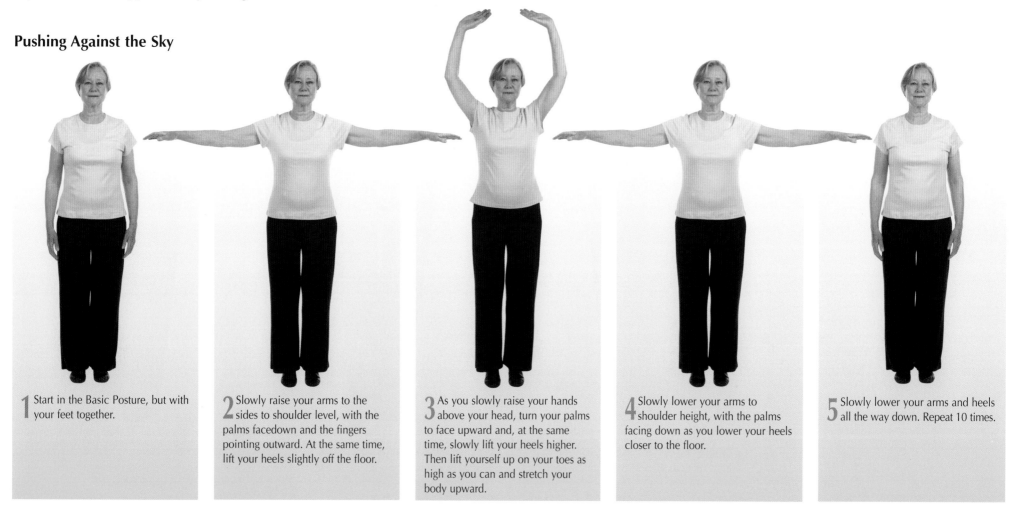

1 Start in the Basic Posture, but with your feet together.

2 Slowly raise your arms to the sides to shoulder level, with the palms facedown and the fingers pointing outward. At the same time, lift your heels slightly off the floor.

3 As you slowly raise your hands above your head, turn your palms to face upward and, at the same time, slowly lift your heels higher. Then lift yourself up on your toes as high as you can and stretch your body upward.

4 Slowly lower your arms to shoulder height, with the palms facing down as you lower your heels closer to the floor.

5 Slowly lower your arms and heels all the way down. Repeat 10 times.

# Simple balancing and strengthening exercise

The Crane Flapping Wings is a good exercise for improving strength as well as balance. If your balance or leg strength is not up to it yet, you can progress in easy stages. First, perform the exercise while lifting only your heel, keeping the toes touching the floor. Later, lift your leg on the upstroke but always lower it to touch the floor on the downstroke. Eventually, keep your leg off the floor through all the repetitions.

To improve strength, perform the exercise slowly. As your strength increases, perform it very slowly. If you wish, you can pause in the low position and hold it for a while for each repetition. Your balance and strength will improve within a few weeks—start with several repetitions and gradually work up to 10 or 20.

## FOLLOW THESE TIPS

- Move your arms up and down as if they are big wings. Pretend you can feel a resistance of the air on your wings.

- Raise and lower your body very slowly—your supporting leg should be moving when your hands are moving.

- Keep good balance throughout and do not let your supporting ankle wobble.

## Crane Flapping Wings

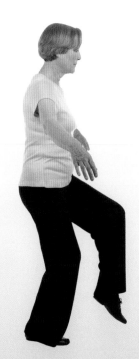

**1** Start in the Basic Posture, but with your feet together. Sink your weight into the right leg as you bend the right knee. Lift up the left heel.

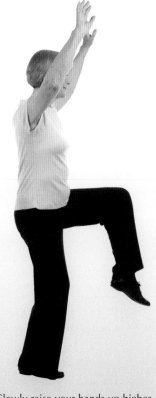

**2** Slowly raise your arms to the sides to waist level, with palms facing down. At the same time, lift your left foot off the floor.

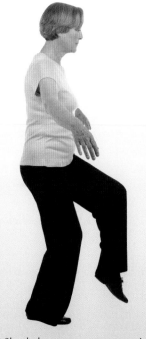

**3** Slowly raise your hands up higher than the head, lifting your fingers to point upward. At the same time, straighten your right leg and lift your left knee higher than your hip.

**4** Slowly lower your arms to waist level with palms facing down as you bend the right knee and lower the left foot near the floor.
Repeat 10 times, then repeat 10 times with the right leg.

# Inner tranquillity and sense of well-being

Your happiness and well-being come from within. You are as much in charge of your mind as you are in charge of your body. Of course, you cannot achieve happiness just by wishing for it. But neither can you change your balance just by wishing. You need to practice. Hopefully, once you have begun practicing Tai Chi, you will see the results for yourself.

Your body awareness will grow during the initial stages of your Tai Chi practice, and with continued practice your awareness of your mind will grow, too. Change is difficult, but awareness can make it happen. For example, when you become aware of tension in your shoulders, it is difficult to ignore it. Some tension will dissolve as soon as you become aware of it. Some will be more persistent and may be difficult to lose. This is usually because it is more deep-seated and your awareness is just brushing its surface. With deeper awareness, it may be possible to eradicate it more easily.

In today's fast-changing world, inner peace and tranquillity are rare commodities. Our minds are constantly active, stimulated by a multitude of images. Yet even now we can attain and enjoy an oasis of calm. When you have learned the Form and practiced it for a time, you will be able to enter a world of slow, graceful movement where your breathing becomes soft and quiet and your mind peaceful.

Tai Chi will improve your ability to relax, your concentration, your balance, your coordination, your strength, your ability to cope with stress, and your health. All these will add up to an increased sense of well-being and confidence, a greater enjoyment of life, and a longer one as well!

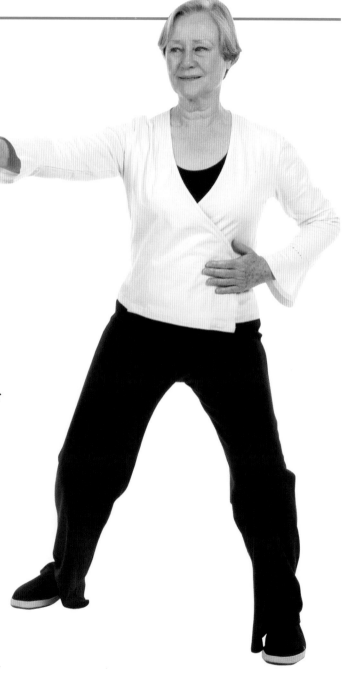

## TAI CHI BENEFITS THAT LEAD TO A SENSE OF WELL-BEING

Practicing Tai Chi regularly will help you:

- Relax better
- Increase your concentration
- Improve your balance
- Achieve better coordination
- Gain greater strength
- Increase your confidence
- Cope better with stress
- Sleep better
- Enjoy better health
- Take pleasure in life

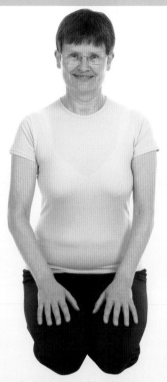

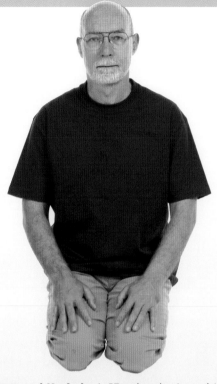

The models in this book are teachers or students of Tai Chi, or both. All find Tai Chi an invaluable source of health and well-being and look forward to keeping Tai Chi a part of their everyday life. Their continued enthusiasm for Tai Chi is an inspiration for those thinking of taking it up.

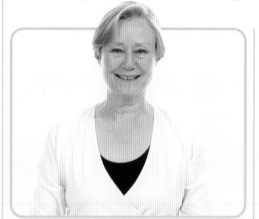

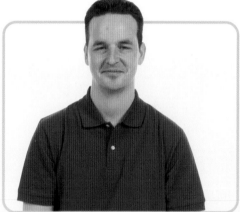

*"Tai Chi gives me the stamina to teach full-time and keep up with my energetic grandchildren."*

*"One of the main benefits of Tai Chi is that it's an antidote to the stress of a professional life."*

**E**va Koskuba is 56 and has been studying Internal Martial Arts since 1982 and teaching since 1986. Her main teacher was her husband Karel, but she also studies with Masters Chen Xiaowang and Du Xianming (still going strong at 87 in Beijing). She and her husband regularly visit China to further their Tai Chi Chuan studies. In March 2006 Eva was accepted as a lineage disciple (twentieth-generation Chen style) by Master Chen Xiaowang.

Eva actively pursues the health and meditative aspects as well as the martial side of the Chinese Internal Martial Arts and different styles of Qigong. With her student Dawn Hatton, a retired nurse, she set up the Tai Chi exercises program for the Battle Hospital in the U.K.

She is looking forward to many more years of practicing, improving, and teaching Tai Chi.

**K**arel Koskuba is 57 and teaches Internal Arts in Berkshire in Britain full-time. He also leads seminars in the U.K. and abroad. He has been studying Internal Martial Arts since 1978 and teaching since 1984. In March 2006 Karel was accepted as a lineage disciple (twentieth-generation Chen style) by Master Chen Xiaowang.

Karel has become deeply interested in mind-body interaction and the impact the practice of Internal Arts has on our body, health, personality, and mind. He has observed—on himself and others—how the practice of Tai Chi slowly improves both the body and the mind.

**K**athy Webb is in her sixties and is a full-time Tai Chi and Qigong teacher. She has practiced Tai Chi since 1988 and became interested in Tai Chi while still a Yoga teacher. Unable to perform many Yoga postures following an accident, she found that Tai Chi was better suited to her body.

Kathy's Tai Chi students include teenage boys at Eton College, an elite private preparatory school; members of the Women's Institute of Great Britain, some in their late seventies and eighties; and people of all ages and abilities at sport and health centers.

She is indebted to her teachers, Eva and Karel Koskuba, but has been particularly inspired by Master Chen Xiaowang, who visits the U.K. every year.

Kathy's ambition is to raise people's awareness of the benefits of Tai Chi.

**J**ohn Henry is 33 and practices law in Great Britain. He has been studying Tai Chi for six years.

John's original interest in Tai Chi came from his involvement with martial arts. He had been studying Karate for six years and found that it was damaging his body, so Tai Chi seemed to be the ideal substitute.

Although John retains an interest in the martial arts, he finds that Tai Chi movements work very deep inside the body to release tensions that have built up and that their calming nature brings back some of the balance that is lost during a day in the office.

John believes that practicing Tai Chi in the mornings before work is particularly beneficial because it enables him to start the day on the right note.

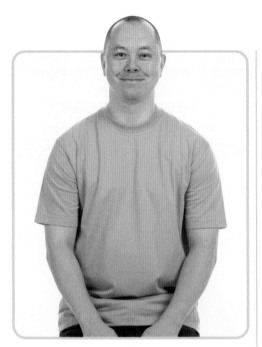

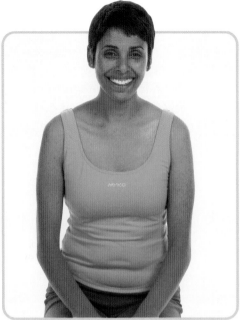

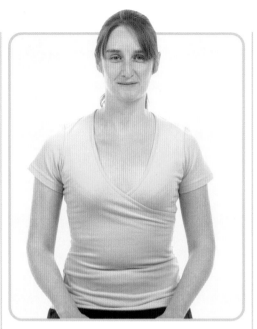

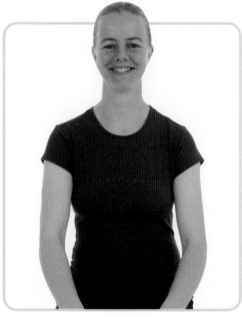

*"The longer I study Tai Chi, the more complex it becomes, but you can take it to whatever level you want."*

*"Tai Chi is the chance to take responsibility for your own health."*

*"I chose Tai Chi because it promotes strength and flexibility in different areas of the body."*

*"Tai Chi is valuable because it builds strength and at the same time increases relaxation."*

**G**avin Wong is 38 and is a police officer in Great Britain. He had always been interested in Tai Chi, but it wasn't until five years ago that he finally had the courage to try it out. He has been practicing ever since.

Gavin wasn't quite sure what to expect when he started studying Tai Chi, but now finds that it is an excellent form of exercise. "It's something you can practice every day without having to go to a gym, and you don't need expensive equipment or clothing."

Gavin considers that Tai Chi fits well into his lifestyle because he can practice at any time of the day. He wants to develop the internal strength aspects of Tai Chi and hopefully to start teaching as well.

**A**mritah Lutchanah is a 30-year-old complementary medicine practitioner. She had always been interested in Tai Chi and eventually started lessons because she felt that it would benefit her general health and well-being.

Amritah has been practicing Tai Chi for two years now, and it has made her much more relaxed. Her practice has also helped enormously to alleviate the effects of the muscle fatigue from which she suffers.

Because Tai Chi has proved so beneficial, Amritah makes the time in her busy day to practice first thing in the morning and again in the evening.

**A**lison Davidson is 27 years old and has been working in an office environment for the past five years but is currently looking for a less sedentary job.

Alison started Tai Chi classes about three years ago when she was looking for something to complement her Yiquan, which she had already been doing for about two years. The fact that the Form could be broken down into sections and used as short exercises in their own right appealed to her. The main reason Alison enjoys Tai Chi, however, is because the movements are quite challenging.

Because Tai Chi promotes strength, flexibility, and power, it is particularly useful for the improvement of her martial arts skills in Yiquan. When Alison was working at a desk job, she also discovered that practicing Tai Chi was a very good way to destress—once she started concentrating on the Form, she would forget all about work!

**E**mma Westlake is 36 years old and has been practicing Tai Chi for 14 years. She teaches several Tai Chi classes a week.

When Emma first started to practice Tai Chi, she was suffering from digestive problems; Tai Chi was a form of exercise she could do that was gentle but still effective. She believes that it supports everything that she does, and it gives a good grounding to her work as a craniosacral therapist.

Teaching Tai Chi has been very rewarding for Emma, and she loves the friendly and supportive atmosphere that develops in her classes. She has found it particularly inspiring to see her over-60 students build and maintain their strength and mobility.

To Emma, Tai Chi is more than just a physical exercise—it is a fascinating study that is good for the mind, body, and spirit.

# GLOSSARY

This glossary is a quick reference for Tai Chi terminology. It covers the terms that will be helpful for Tai Chi students and provides pronounciation where useful.

## Spelling Chinese words

There are a number of ways to transliterate Chinese using the Latin alphabet. The spellings in this book are those that are the most familiar to English speakers. Some spellings follow the older, better-known system called Wade-Giles, and others the newer system called Pinyin. (This glossary gives the most popular current spelling, followed by the alternative.)

In the Wade-Giles system, apostrophes originally played an important role in distinguishing "hard" and "soft" consonants—for example, in the spelling T'ai Chi Ch'uan. These were often used incorrectly and were increasingly omitted altogether.

Wade-Giles spellings are gradually being abandoned in favor of the simpler Pinyin system, which has been officially adopted by the Chinese government and is gaining worldwide acceptance. Street signs in Beijing are now written in Pinyin as well as Chinese characters. Pinyin more accurately reflects the pronunciation of Chinese words, but unfortunately for English speakers, it is based on French pronunciation. The Wade-Giles use of "ch" is replaced in Pinyin by j, q, or zh. Another obvious difference is that the Wade-Giles system writes each Chinese character separately, whereas in Pinyin the sounds are combined into one word—for example, T'ai Chi Ch'uan becomes Taijiquan.

**an**
One of the four main techniques or energies of Tai Chi; in Pushing Hands it is used to press down and forward.

**Baguazhang (Pa Kua Chang)**
[pronounced *ba gua zhang*] Eight Trigram Palm Boxing; a Chinese internal martial art whose characteristics are the use of evasion and circling.

**Basic Posture**
Same balanced standing position as the Basic Stance.

**Basic Stance**
Tai Chi standing position with the feet shoulder-width apart and the weight distributed evenly between the feet.

**Central Equilibrium**
The quality of being balanced in all directions; a necessary condition for the development of internal power in Tai Chi.

**chansi jin (chan ssu chin)**
[pronounced *chan s' tchin*] See Silk Reeling.

**Chen-Style Tai Chi**
One of the main styles of Tai Chi, distinguished by its use of Silk Reeling. Considered the first style to have been developed.

**chi (qi)**
[pronounced *chee*] A generic term that is used for many phenomena. In Tai Chi it is most often used to mean breath, intrinsic energy, or the coordination of body by intent.

**dantian (tan tien)**
[pronounced *dan tien*] Anatomically the center of gravity in the body. In Daoism it is "the field of cinnabar." Human *chi* is said to originate here, since all movement is preceded by stabilization of the lower back.

**Dao (Tao)**
[pronounced *dow*] The Way; as well as the big Dao—the Way of Nature and Universe—every person and every activity has its own (small) Dao.

**Dao De Jing (Tao Te Ching)**
[pronounced *dow d' tching*] The Way and its Virtue; the first classic of Daoism attributed to Lao Zi.

**Daoism (Taoism)**
Daoism is one of the three great philosophies of China (Buddhism and Confucianism are the other two). It seeks balance in everything by following the Dao.

**daoyin (tao yin)**
Guiding and leading the *chi* using first breath and later the mind. A precursor of Qigong.

**double weighting**
This term refers to any number of errors in one's posture that impair the freedom of movement and are caused by not taking into account the flow of forces through the body (usually a result of lack of awareness). The name comes from the most common type of posture error: incorrect distribution of the body's weight.

**essential softness/hardness**
Two qualities of the body that are necessary for developing internal power in Tai Chi. First, one must develop essential softness by getting rid of all unnecessary tension, both in standing and moving (*see also* song). Only then can one develop essential hardness.

**fajin (fa chin)**
[pronounced *fa tchin*] Release of energy or strength, usually as a fast, explosive movement; the prerequisite for developing fajin is achieving essential softness.

**Form, the Tai Chi**
A series of Tai Chi movements linked together to create an exercise routine that is used for the practice of Tai Chi. Each Tai Chi style has a Form of its own, or several. "Form" can also be used to describe a movement within a complete Form.

**full/empty**
Another name for substantial/ insubstantial.

**hardness, essential**
*See* essential softness/hardness.

**inguinal crease**
The area of the body in the groin where a diagonal crease is formed when the leg is rotated at the hip. *See also* kua.

**insubstantial**
*See* substantial/insubstantial.

**internal connection**
In Tai Chi the body is internally connected if it forms a cohesive unit that is not dependent on using phasic muscles. Instead, it relies on stabilizing muscles, fascia, tendons, and ligaments.

**internal martial arts**
Internal martial arts uses the mind in developing strength, unlike external martial arts (such as wrestling, boxing, karate), which rely mainly on physical strength training. The three main Chinese internal martial arts are Xingyiquan, Baguazhang, and Tai Chi Chuan. They all focus on cultivating intrinsic energy (*chi*) and on fighting methods based on using the opponent's strength against them.

**internal power**
*See* neijin.

**ji (chee)**
[pronounced *tchee*] One of the four main techniques or energies of Tai Chi; in Pushing Hands it is used to push forward.

**jin (chin)**
[pronounced *tchin*] Refined, skilled strength, which is the fusion of *chi* and strength. Often used as a synonym of neijin.

**kua (gua)**
[pronounced *gwa*] The area of the body where the leg meets the body; it includes the hip joint and associated muscles and connective tissue. Sometimes it refers only to the inguinal crease.

**li**
[pronounced *lih*] Strength; when contrasted with jin, it means untrained, clumsy strength.

# Glossary

**lu**
One of the four main techniques or energies of Tai Chi; in Pushing Hands it is used to redirect incoming push.

***mingmen***
An acupuncture point in the middle of the lower back (between the 2nd and 3rd lumbar vertebrae).

**muscles—phasic and tonic**
These terms are used in this book to explain correct muscle use in Tai Chi. Phasic refers to muscles when they respond to our conscious control, also called mobilizers. Tonic refers to muscles that are used outside of our volition, mainly to support and stabilize our body, also called fixators, stabilizers, or postural muscles.
   One muscle can be in both the phasic and tonic categories depending on usage, but when it is used as a phasic muscle, it has different characteristics in terms of its neural control and its fiber use than when it is used as a stabilizer. In effect, it acts as two different types of muscle.

**Neijia (Nei Chia)**
[pronounced *nee tchia*] A school of internal martial arts.

**neijin (nei chin)**
[pronounced *nee tchin*] Internal power; whole-body power capable of using a springlike strength in any direction.

**open/close**
The Tai Chi principle of coordinating the movement of the body to enhance the whole-body power; during the close phase, predominantly flexors are used; during the open phase, mainly extensors are used.

**peng**
[pronounced *pung*] Springlike quality of the body in Tai Chi; synonymous with internal power, especially when referred to as peng jin. It is also one of the four main techniques or energies of Tai Chi; in Pushing Hands it is used to intercept and neutralize an incoming force.

**peng, lu, ji, an**
The four main techniques or energies of Tai Chi Chuan used in Pushing Hands or combat; meaning to ward off, roll back, push, and press respectively.

**phasic muscles**
*See* muscles—phasic and tonic.

**posture, Tai Chi**
A static configuration of the body that serves some function, usually in learning a movement or training the body or mind.

**Pushing Hands**
Interactive Tai Chi partner exercises designed to practice and train sensitivity, listening, sticking, following, and the main jins (peng, lu, ji, an). Some variations are also used as a bridge to practicing martial

applications—for example, Da Lu. Also called Four Corners Pushing Hands.

**Qigong (Chi Kung)**
[pronounced *chee gung*] Traditional Chinese therapeutic exercises used to cultivate *chi*.

**qinna (chin na)**
[pronounced *chin na*] Seize and control; the name given to a method of controlling an opponent by manipulation (usually quite painful) of joints, muscles, and tendons.

**rooting**
Ability to stick to the ground when pushed or pulled. A measure of how well the center is connected to the foot and how well a force can be directed or led to the ground.

**shen**
[pronounced *shun*] Spirit, strength of mind, will, and courage.

**Silk Reeling**
The coiling/twisting movement of an "internally connected" body (Silk Reeling energy or chansi jin) and the Tai Chi exercises designed to train this type of special movement (Silk Reeling exercises). Silk Reeling motion is the basis of all Chen-Style Tai Chi movement.

**sinking**
Apparent lowering of the center of gravity by relaxing joints (mainly hips and legs).

**Six Harmonies**
Description of the correct conduct of the body and mind in internal martial arts. The Three External Harmonies describe the conduct of the body—shoulders harmonize with hips, elbows with knees, and hands with feet. The Three Internal Harmonies describe how the mind generates strength—desire harmonizes with intent, intent with *chi*, and *chi* with strength.

**softness, essential**
*See* essential softness/hardness.

**song (sung)**
[pronounced *sung*] A state of alert relaxation, often described as the state a cat is in when it is waiting to pounce on a mouse. This state is characterized by all phasic muscles being relaxed and the body supported by postural muscles only; basis of essential softness.

**stance, Tai Chi**
A (usually) simple standing position that is common to a number of Tai Chi postures. Usually related to an action or a movement.

**substantial/insubstantial**
An expression of Yin/Yang in one's body. A point or an area of the body is "substantial" if it is subject to some force (which could be gravity) that it actively resists. "Insubstantial" refers to a point where there is no resistance to a force.

**Tai Chi (Taiji)**
[pronounced *tai tchee*] A shortened, commonly used name for Tai Chi Chuan.

**Tai Chi Chuan (Taijiquan)**
[pronounced *tai tchee chu an*] Literally translated as The Supreme Ultimate Boxing. More accurately translated as Yin/Yang Boxing, since the word Tai Chi is the name of the Yin/Yang symbol (see page 7 for a picture of the symbol).

**Tai Chi *Classics***
A collection of writings containing the fundamental principles of Tai Chi Chuan. Attributed to early Chinese masters of Tai Chi.

**TCM**
This is the acronym for traditional Chinese medicine. Comprehensive system of medicine, including herbal remedies, acupuncture, and therapeutic exercises.

**tonic muscles**
*See* muscles—phasic and tonic.

**Weijia (Wei Chia)**
A school of external martial arts.

**Wuji (Wu Chi)**
[pronounced *wu jee*] Primordial empty state; means extreme emptiness.

**wuwei**
[pronounced *wu way*] Nonaction; achieving one's goal by allowing a natural flow of events to take their course.

***xin* (*hsin*)**
[pronounced *shin*] Mind, heart, or desire.

**Xingyiquan (Hsing I Chuan)**
[pronounced *shing yee chwen*] Form and Intent Boxing; one of the main Chinese internal martial arts.

***yi* (*i*)**
[pronounced *yee*] Mind, will, or intent.

**Yin/Yang**
Traditional Chinese concepts used to explain the nature of reality and all within it as an interaction or relationship of opposing qualities that naturally complement themselves; for example, dark/light, cold/hot, contract/expand, low/high, feminine/masculine, wet/dry, and so on.
   In Tai Chi it is used to refer to weighted/unweighted, passive/active, slow/fast, soft/hard, and so on.

**Yiquan (I Chuan)**
[pronounced *yee chwen*] Intent Boxing; one of the main Chinese internal martial arts.

**Zhan Zhuang**
A Qigong standing practice that enables the *chi* to sink to the *dantian*. Used in internal martial arts to strengthen the body "from within"—to strengthen the function of stabilizers.

# A BRIEF HISTORY OF TAI CHI

Tai Chi is a treasure of Chinese civilization, and there are various myths and legends about its origins. The most popular features a Daoist immortal, Zhang Sangfen, who was said to have created Tai Chi Chuan after observing (or dreaming about) a fight between a snake and a crane.

The theory supported by the most documented evidence, however, is that Tai Chi originated in the Chen Village in the province of Henan during the seventeenth century. Its founder was a Ming military officer, Chen Wangting, who, after retiring from government service, created a new form of martial art, drawing from the rich source of Chinese martial arts and the health cultivation tradition of Daoyin. This new martial art later became known as Tai Chi Chuan, and its unique characteristics helped it evolve into one of the most popular health systems practiced today.

The fundamental principles of Tai Chi come from a collection of writings called the Tai Chi *Classics*, which are attributed to various early masters of the art. The history of Tai Chi is closely bound with the most prominent masters in each generation.

Here is a list of the masters who shaped its evolution:

### Chen Wangting (1600–1680)
Called the Father of Tai Chi Chuan, Chen Wangting was a warrior, a scholar, and a ninth-generation Chen patriarch. He is credited with creating Tai Chi. His style became known as the Chen School. It combines soft and hard, slow and fast, and obvious body spiraling.

### Chen Changxing (1771–1853)
The fourteenth-generation Chen patriarch Chen Changxing gave the Chen-Style Tai Chi Chuan the Form it has today by combining the several sets created by Chen Wangting into a slow set and a fast set (Cannon Fist). He was the first to teach Chen-Style Tai Chi Chuan to an outsider (Yang Luchan).

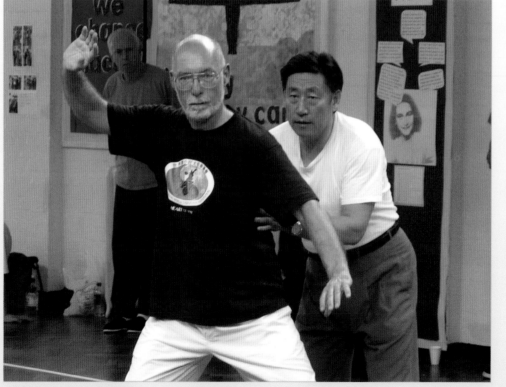

### Yang Luchan (1799–1872)
A student of Chen Changxing and the founder of the Yang School, Yang Luchan based the Yang Form on the first set of the Chen Style (the slow set). Because of his skill, he became known as Yang the Invincible.

### Wu Yuxiang (1812–1880)
Wu Yuxiang was the founder of the Wuu School, also called Hao after Hao Wei Zhen, the second-generation successor of Wu Yuxiang. (The Wuu spelling was adopted to avoid confusion with the Wu Style of Wu Jianquan.) He was a student of Yang Luchan and later went to Chen Village to study with Chen Qingping. The Wuu Style is characterized by compact, rounded, precise, and high-standing postures and is also known as the Old Wu Style.

### Sun Lutang (1861–1932)
Founder of the Sun School, Sun Lutang learned Tai Chi Chuan from Hao Wei Zhen. He developed a new style

Master Chen Xiaowang gives an advanced master class to author Karel Koskuba (foreground). Master Chen is the current head of the Chen Style. He teaches Chen-Style Tai Chi Chuan worldwide.

by combining Tai Chi principles with his knowledge of Baguazhang and Xingyiquan (see Glossary on pages 139 and 140). This style is characterized by high postures with active steps and emphasis on "open and close."

## Wu Jianquan (1870–1942)

Wu Jianquan is the founder of the Wu School. He was taught by his father Quan You, who was an outstanding student of Yang Luchan, and his son Yang Banhou. This style is characterized by small, uniformly slow movements and leaning postures.

## Yang Chengfu (1883–1936)

The grandson of Yang Luchan, Yang Chengfu is reputed to have taught thousands of students and popularized Tai Chi throughout China. The development of the Yang Style culminated with Yang Chengfu, who gave it the appearance we know today—expansive and even movements.

## Chen Fake (1887–1957)

The seventeenth-generation Chen patriarch Chen Fake brought the Chen Style from the Chen Village to Beijing and is credited with creating the New Style (Xinjia).

## Chen Xiaowang (1946– )

The nineteenth-generation Chen patriarch and the current head of the Chen Style, Chen Xiaowang has taught many thousands of students worldwide. He has done for Chen Style on a world scale what Yang Chengfu had accomplished for Yang Style in China. Apart from Tai Chi, Master Chen's other passion is calligraphy (see below). Both Tai Chi and calligraphy involve the same transportation of *chi* (*yu qi*) in our body to the point of action.

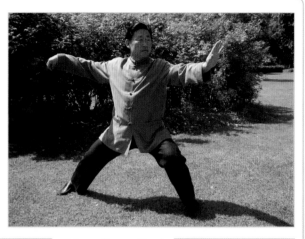

Right: Master Chen Xiaowang, the current head of the Chen Style, demonstrates Tai Chi in a park.

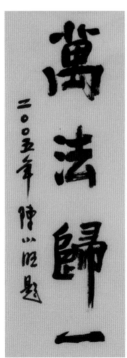

This scroll drawn by Master Chen Xiaowang says: "Ten thousand techniques return to one." Ten thousand is the Chinese way of saying "many, many," and "return" means "return to the source/origin."

Therefore, it means that the various techniques used in Tai Chi all come from one principle, and as one progresses in Tai Chi, it becomes evident that all the techniques may have different Forms but really they are still just taken from one principle.

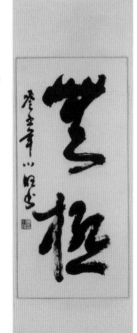

Master Chen wrote on this scroll "Wu Ji," or "extreme emptiness." Wuji is represented by an empty circle.

According to Chinese legend, Wuji is the state of the universe before anything was there. Later something moved and the emptiness divided into Yin and Yang (Tai Chi); the interaction of Yin and Yang gave rise to everything else. Hence the Chinese saying: "Wuji is the mother of Tai Chi and Tai Chi is the mother of all things."

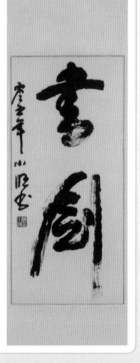

This scroll says: "Book and sword." It means that it is important both to study theory (the book) and to practice (applications).

The book represents a scholar, and the sword represents a warrior. Master Chen's advice here is that to be good at Tai Chi, you need to be a combination of both.

142

# Index

# Index—continued